Procedure Notes for Interventional Pain Medicine Fellows

Procedure Notes for Interventional Pain Medicine Fellows

By

K. C. Maasumi and Sam Scire

Cambridge Scholars Publishing

Procedure Notes for Interventional Pain Medicine Fellows

By K. C. Maasumi and Sam Scire

This book first published 2023

Cambridge Scholars Publishing

Lady Stephenson Library, Newcastle upon Tyne, NE6 2PA, UK

British Library Cataloguing in Publication Data
A catalogue record for this book is available from the British Library

ISBN (10): 1-5275-2860-X
ISBN (13): 978-1-5275-2860-4

I dedicate this book to my wife who stood by my side
through hard times,
to my parents who helped me immigrate to this amazing country
in hope of prosperity,
and to my son who has brought joy to my life.

—K. C. Maasumi

TABLE OF CONTENTS

INTRODUCTION

The discipline of pain medicine is complex and fascinating. It reaches out to a variety of medical disciplines in order to provide a comprehensive treatment for patients. Pain is generally defined as a localized or generalized unpleasant bodily sensation or complex of sensations that causes mild to severe physical discomfort and emotional distress. Therefore, in order to treat pain properly, a provider has to utilize their knowledge from orthopedics, psychology, anatomy, neurology and more. Since we all come from different disciplines, it is very important to collaborate with our colleagues and know our limitations. We often use interventional pain management techniques to alleviate pain temporarily. This provides a window of opportunity for the patient to utilize other modalities to help with the pain including but not limited to physical therapy, which helps strengthen the muscles surrounding the painful body parts. As basic sciences in pain medicine progress, we may utilize more specific molecular treatments focused on the painful areas to alleviate the pain.

The purpose of this book is to provide you with a glimpse of how a typical intervention can be performed. Please know, this is just a template and the details on how the procedure is actually performed is in the hand of the practitioner and remains your responsibility. This book does not cover all the possible procedures, their variations, nor does it replace a fellowship in pain medicine. This is a collection of procedures that are commonly performed by interventional pain providers whose experience and knowledge dictates the probable outcome of the procedure. Performing a procedure is a team effort. Depending on the complexity of the procedure, several people may be involved including but not limited to the interventional pain physician, radiological technologist and nursing staff. Communication with radiologic technologist is very crucial and helpful to the flow of the procedure which can aid in achieving favorable outcomes.

Fluoroscopy (C-arm) is the most common imaging modality used in interventional pain management. The true benefit of utilizing a C-arm during interventional pain procedures is the ability to alter the angle to better define the pathway to the target. The practitioner advances the needle in the same parallel plane(s) as the angle and obliquity of the C-arm. Frequently adjustments to the angles are very minute for optimal identification of the anatomy and the pathway to the target point. Proper protection against radiation, practicing safe distance, reducing fluoroscopy-time, and proper shielding should be practiced reducing exposure.

CHAPTER 1

HEAD & NECK PROCEDURES

K.C. MAASUMI, M.D., M.S.

List of procedures in this chapter:

- Gasserian/Trigeminal Ganglion Block
- Gasserian Ganglion Radiofrequency Ablation under Fluoroscopy
- Supraorbital and Supratrochlear Nerve Block
- Supraorbital Nerve Radio Frequency Ablation with Ultrasound Guidance
- Temporo-auricular Nerve Block
- Greater and Lesser Occipital Nerve Block
- Occipital Nerve Block under Ultrasound Guidance
- Radiofrequency Ablation of Greater Occipital Nerves
- Sphenopalatine Ganglion Block
- OnabotulinumtoxinA Injections (PREEMPT Protocol)

Procedure name: Gasserian/Trigeminal Ganglion Block

Diagnosis:

Consent: The risks, benefits and anticipated outcomes of the procedure, the risks and benefits of the alternatives to the procedure, and the roles and tasks of the personnel involved, were discussed with the patient. The patient has given written informed consent to the procedure and agrees to proceed.

Anesthesia:

Attending physician:

Assisting physician:

Patient information:

Procedure details: The patient was brought into the procedure room and placed in the supine position on the fluoroscopy table. Standard monitors were placed, and vital signs were observed throughout the procedure. The patient's affected side of the face was prepped and draped in a sterile manner. Fluoroscopic views of the foramen ovale were optimized with oblique angulation in a submental trajectory. The skin and subcutaneous tissues over the intended trajectory, 2 cm lateral to the apex of the mouth, were anesthetized. A 3.5-inch, 22-gauge spinal needle was inserted through the anesthetized skin towards the foramen ovale in a coaxial fashion under fluoroscopic guidance. Intermittent lateral views were obtained to assess the depth of the needle tip. Proper depth of the spinal needle was confirmed with the needle tip just into the foramen ovale at the junction of the posterior clinoid process and the skull base. After negative aspiration, contrast was injected with spread along the foramen ovale, without vascular uptake. After repeat aspiration, 2 cc of a mixture composed of 1 cc of ropivacaine 0.5%, and 1 cc of 10mg/ml dexamethasone preservative free was injected in a slow incremental fashion while monitoring the patient's response. The needle stylet was replaced, and the needle was removed with the tip intact.

Disposition: The patient tolerated the procedure well without apparent complications. The patient was able to ambulate out of the facility in the same fashion they had entered. Discharge instructions were given.

Procedure name: Gasserian Ganglion Radiofrequency Ablation under Fluoroscopy

Diagnosis:

Consent: The risks, benefits and anticipated outcomes of the procedure, the risks and benefits of the alternatives to the procedure, and the roles and tasks of the personnel involved, were discussed with the patient. The patient has given written informed consent to the procedure and agrees to proceed.

Anesthesia:

Attending physician:

Assisting physician:

Patient information:

Procedure detail: The patient was brought to the procedure room and positioned supine on the fluoroscopy table. A 27-gauge peripheral IV was inserted and intravenous fluid was provided prior to the start of the procedure. Standard monitors were placed, and vital signs were observed throughout the procedure. The patient's affected side of the face was prepped and draped in a sterile manner. Fluoroscopic views of the foramen ovale were optimized with oblique angulation in a submental trajectory. At a location 2 cm lateral to the apex of the mouth, the skin and subcutaneous tissues over the intended trajectory were anesthetized. A radiofrequency needle was inserted through the anesthetized skin towards the foramen ovale in a coaxial fashion under fluoroscopic guidance. Intermittent lateral views were obtained to assess the depth of the needle tip. Proper depth of the spinal needle confirmed with the needle tip just into the foramen ovale at the junction of the posterior clinoid process and the skull base.

Sensory testing was done once the needle tip was deemed to be in the correct location with patient reporting sensation in the right upper and lower lip. Motor testing showed masseter muscle pulsation. Pulsed radiofrequency ablation at 42 degrees Celsius for 120 seconds was performed with the needle tip pointing medially. Ablation was repeated a few times, each time turning the tip of the needle 90 degrees. Contrast was injected to ensure that there is not any vascular uptake. Then 0.5 cc of 10 mg/ml dexamethasone was injected. The needle was then removed after being restyletted with the tip intact. There was appropriate paresthesia in the affected trigeminal nerve distribution.

Disposition: The patient tolerated the procedure well without apparent complications. The patient was able to ambulate out of the facility in the same fashion they had entered. Discharge instructions were given.

Procedure name: Supraorbital and Supratrochlear Nerve Block

Diagnosis:

Consent: The risks, benefits and anticipated outcomes of the procedure, the risks and benefits of the alternatives to the procedure, and the roles and tasks of the personnel involved, were discussed with the patient. The patient has given written informed consent to the procedure and agrees to proceed.

Anesthesia:

Attending physician:

Assisting physician:

Patient information:

Procedure detail: The area of injection was identified above the plane of the affected eyebrow. The area was cleaned and prepped in sterile fashion. A 1-inch 30-gauge hypodermic needle was attached to a 1 cc syringe. The needle was inserted into the dermis and directed medially, parallel and above the glabella to a point passing slightly the vertical plane of the ipsilateral pupil. Aspiration ensured the injection is not intravascular. The injectate was slowly given; as the injection continued, the needle was gently withdrawn to cover the supratrochlear nerve.

Disposition: The patient tolerated the procedure well without apparent complications. Patient was able to ambulate out of the facility in the same fashion they had entered. Discharge instructions were given.*

---

* NOTE: This procedure can also be done using ultrasound. A linear ultrasound probe is draped with a sterile probe cover. Sonographic examination with sterile sonographic gel is utilized to reveal supraorbital ridge. A 27ga 1.5-inch needle is advanced with ultrasound guidance until the needle tip is visualized to advance to the supraorbital foramen. Once negative aspiration is confirmed, the injectate was given.

Procedure name: Supraorbital Nerve Radio Frequency Ablation with Ultrasound Guidance

Diagnosis:

Consent: The risks, benefits and anticipated outcomes of the procedure, the risks and benefits of the alternatives to the procedure, and the roles and tasks of the personnel involved, were discussed with the patient. The patient has given written informed consent to the procedure and agrees to proceed.

Anesthesia:

Attending physician:

Assisting physician:

Patient information:

Procedure details: The patient was brought to the procedure room and placed in the supine position on the fluoroscopy table. Proper support was provided under the head to make patient comfortable. Standard monitors were placed, and vital signs were observed throughout the procedure. The area of the forehead was prepped and draped in a sterile manner. A linear ultrasound probe was draped with a sterile probe cover. Sonographic examination with sterile sonographic gel revealed supraorbital foramen. The skin and subcutaneous tissues at the targeted point were anesthetized with 1% lidocaine. A 22ga radiofrequency needle was advanced with ultrasound guidance until the needle tip landed over the supraorbital foramen. Then after sensory testing at 1.5V, pulsed radiofrequency ablation was carried out for 2 minutes. This step can be repeated as deemed appropriate.

Disposition: The patient tolerated the procedure well without apparent complications. The patient was able to ambulate out of the facility in the same fashion they had entered. Discharge instructions were given.

Procedure name: Temporo-auricular Nerve Block

Diagnosis:

Consent: The risks, benefits and anticipated outcomes of the procedure, the risks and benefits of the alternatives to the procedure, and the roles and tasks of the personnel involved, were discussed with the patient. The patient has given written informed consent to the procedure and agrees to proceed.

Anesthesia:

Attending physician:

Assisting physician:

Patient information:

Procedure details: The area of injection was identified as the affected anterior tragus. The auriculo-temporal artery was palpated and identified. The area was cleaned draped in a sterile fashion. A 30-gauge 0.5-inch hypodermic needle was attached to a 1 cc syringe. The needle was inserted just deep to the dermis and pushed superior and posteriorly and advanced for 1 cm. Aspiration ensured lack of intravascular injection. 1 cc of the 0.5% bupivacaine mixed with 1 cc of 10m/ml dexamethasone was used to inject 1-2 cc of the mixture and the needle was slowly withdrawn with the tip intact.

Disposition: The patient tolerated the procedure well without apparent complications. The patient was able to ambulate out of the facility in the same fashion they had entered. Discharge instructions were given.

Procedure name: Greater and Lesser Occipital Nerve Block

Diagnosis:

Consent: The risks, benefits and anticipated outcomes of the procedure, the risks and benefits of the alternatives to the procedure, and the roles and tasks of the personnel involved, were discussed with the patient. The patient has given written informed consent to the procedure and agrees to proceed.

Anesthesia:

Attending physician:

Assisting physician:

Patient information:

Procedure detail: The patient was brought into the procedure room and placed in a seated position. The occipital artery was palpated and the point of maximal tenderness lateral to the artery was identified for the blockade of the greater occipital nerve. This area was prepped and cleaned. A 27-gauge, 1.25-inch needle was inserted into the dermis. Care was taken not to contact the occipital bone. Negative aspiration was confirmed and a subcutaneous deposition of 1-3 cc of a mixture of 1 cc of 1% lidocaine, 1 cc of 0.5% bupivacaine and 1 cc of 10mg/ml dexamethasone was injected. The needle was then removed with the tip intact.

Attention was directed toward injecting the lesser occipital nerve. The inion and the mastoid process was palpated. A location 1/3 the distance between the mastoid process and the inion was chosen medial to the mastoid process. Again, a 27-gauge, 1.5-inch hypodermic needle was used to inject 1-2 cc of the same mixture above.

Disposition: Patient tolerated the procedure well without apparent complications. Patient was able to ambulate out of the facility in the same fashion they had entered. Discharge instructions were given.

Procedure name: Occipital Nerve Block under Ultrasound Guidance

Diagnosis:

Consent: The risks, benefits and anticipated outcomes of the procedure, the risks and benefits of the alternatives to the procedure, and the roles and tasks of the personnel involved, were discussed with the patient. The patient has given written informed consent to the procedure and agrees to proceed.

Anesthesia:

Attending physician:

Assisting physician:

Patient information:

Procedure detail: The patient was brought into the procedure room and placed in a prone position on the procedure table. C2 spinous process was identified under ultrasound visualization. Scanning laterally revealed the trapezius, semispinalis capitis, and inferior oblique capitis muscles. An ellipsoid hyperechoic structure between the inferior oblique and semispinalis was identified as the greater occipital nerve approximately 2 cm deep in the skin. After identifying the proper location, the area was prepped and draped in a sterile fashion. A 30-gauge, 1-inch needle was used to anesthetize the skin and subcutaneous tissue. Then, a curved probe covered with sterile ultrasound cover was used to guide a 23-gauge, 3.5-inch spinal needle in an out-of-plane approach to the identified location. If needed, incremental tissue dissection was used to identify the tip of the needle. Negative aspiration was confirmed, and 1-2 cc of a mixture consisting of 1 cc of 0.5% bupivacaine and 1 cc of 10mg/ml dexamethasone was injected. The needle was then removed with the tip intact.

Disposition: The patient tolerated the procedure well without apparent complications. The patient was able to ambulate out of the facility in the same fashion they had entered. Discharge instructions were given.

Procedure name: Radiofrequency Ablation of Greater Occipital Nerves

Diagnosis:

Consent: The risks, benefits and anticipated outcomes of the procedure, the risks and benefits of the alternatives to the procedure, and the roles and tasks of the personnel involved, were discussed with the patient. The patient has given written informed consent to the procedure and agrees to proceed.

Anesthesia:

Attending physician:

Assisting physician:

Patient information:

Procedure detail: The patient was brought into the procedure room and placed in a prone position on the procedure table. The occipital artery was palpated and the point of maximal tenderness lateral to the artery was identified. This area was prepped and draped in a sterile fashion. A 2-inch radiofrequency (RF) needle was used to insert medial to the palpated occipital artery. Care was taken not to touch the occipital bone. The stimulator probe was inserted through the RF needle. Using stimulation, a proper location was achieved. Pulsed radiofrequency ablation treatment was initiated with an RF generator using the following parameters:

Voltage output: Usually between 40V and 60V
Frequency: 2 Hz
Pulses: 20 ms pulses in a 1-second cycle
Duration: 120 second per cycle
Impedance: can range between 150 and 400 Ω
Temperature: 42°C
Number of cycles: 3 cycles with slight adjustments of the electrodes (i.e., 45° clockwise, then 45° counterclockwise).
The stimulator was removed, keeping the RF needle in place.
1 cc solution composed of 1 cc of 10mg/ml dexamethasone and 1 cc of 1% lidocaine was used to inject.

Disposition: The patient tolerated the procedure well without apparent complications. The patient was able to ambulate out of the facility in the same fashion they had entered. Discharge instructions were given.

Procedure name: Sphenopalatine Ganglion Block

Diagnosis:

Consent: The risks, benefits and anticipated outcomes of the procedure, the risks and benefits of the alternatives to the procedure, and the roles and tasks of the personnel involved, were discussed with the patient. The patient has given written informed consent to the procedure and agrees to proceed.

Anesthesia:

Attending physician:

Assisting physician:

Patient information:

Procedure detail: The patient was brought into the procedure room and placed in a supine position with the head slightly extended. The area was cleaned and prepped in sterile fashion. Using fluoroscopy, the mandibular nerve 1-2 mm past the posterosuperior border relative to the lateral pterygoid plate OR the maxillary nerve 1-2 mm past the AP border toward the pterygomaxillary fissure were chosen. These landmarks were confirmed using lateral views. A 22-gauge 3.5-inch spinal needle was advanced toward the respective border of the pterygoid plate. Once contact was made with the lateral pterygoid plate, the tip of the needle was walked off 1-2 mm inferiorly. In the AP view, the tip of the needle should lie at the edge of the medial orbital line. Contrast was used to confirm proper placement. 1-2 cc of mixture consisting of 1 cc of 10mg/ml dexamethasone and 1 cc of 0.25% bupivacaine was injected.

Disposition: The patient tolerated the procedure well without apparent complications. The patient was able to ambulate out of the facility in the same fashion they had entered. Discharge instructions were given.

Procedure name: OnabotulinumtoxinA Injections (PREEMPT Protocol)

Diagnosis:

Consent: The risks, benefits and anticipated outcomes of the procedure, the risks and benefits of the alternatives to the procedure, and the roles and tasks of the personnel involved, were discussed with the patient. The patient has given written informed consent to the procedure and agrees to proceed.

Anesthesia:

Attending physician:

Assisting physician:

Patient information:

Procedure detail:

Lot #:
Expiration date:
Diluent: Normal saline 0.9%

Injection Sites

Muscle	Total units	Number of sites	Left	Right
Corrugator	10	2	5	5
Procerus	5	1		
Frontalis	20	4	10	10
Temporalis	40	8	20	20
Occipitalis	30	6	15	15
Cervical paraspinal muscles	20	4	10	10
Trapezius	30	6	15	15
Total	155	31		

Disposition: The patient tolerated the procedure well without apparent complications. The patient was able to ambulate out of the facility in the same fashion they had entered. Discharge instructions were given.

CHAPTER 2

CERVICAL PROCEDURES

SAM SCIRE, R.T., (R)(CT), ARRT, CRT
AND K.C. MAASUMI, M.D., M.S.

List of procedures in this chapter:

- Cervical Interlaminar Epidural Steroid Injection (CESI)
- Cervical Transforaminal Epidural Steroid Injection (TFESI)
- Cervical Selective Nerve Root Block (SNRB)
- Cervical Intra-articular Facet Joint Injection
- Cervical Medial Branch Blocks (MBB)
- Radiofrequency of Cervical Medial Branches
- Cervical Discography

Procedure name: Cervical Interlaminar Epidural Steroid Injection (CESI)

Diagnosis:

Consent: The risks, benefits and anticipated outcomes of the procedure, the risks and benefits of the alternatives to the procedure, and the roles and tasks of the personnel involved, were discussed with the patient. The patient has given written informed consent to the procedure and agrees to proceed.

Anesthesia:

Attending physician:

Assisting physician:

Patient information:

Procedure detail: The patient was transported into the procedure room and was positioned prone on the fluoroscopy table. Monitors were placed and vital signs were observed throughout the procedure. The patient's neck and upper back were prepped and draped in a sterile manner. Using AP and contralateral views, an 22-gauge Touhy epidural needle with an attached loss of resistance syringe was advanced in a coaxial fashion until the ligamentum flavum was engaged and loss of resistance was attained. After negative aspiration to rule out vascular return, contrast was injected under live fluoroscopy demonstrating epidural spread without vascular uptake. 2-5 cc of a mixture of 1 ml of 10mg/ml dexamethasone and 1 cc of 1% lidocaine and normal saline was injected into the epidural space. The needle was then removed, and hemostasis was achieved.

Disposition: Patient tolerated the procedure well without apparent complications. Patient was able to ambulate out of the facility in the same fashion they had entered. Discharge instructions were given.

Procedure name: Cervical Transforaminal Epidural Steroid Injection (TFESI)

Diagnosis:

Consent: The risks, benefits and anticipated outcomes of thc procedure, the risks and benefits of the alternatives to the procedure, and the roles and tasks of the personnel involved, were discussed with the patient. The patient has given written informed consent to the procedure and agrees to proceed.

Anesthesia:

Attending physician:

Assisting physician:

Patient information:

Procedure detail: The patient was transported into the procedure room and was positioned supine on the fluoroscopy table. A time out was performed per the usual clinical fashion. Monitors were placed and vital signs were observed throughout the procedure. The patient's neck was prepped and draped in a sterile manner. The patient's head was turned away from the affected side. The C-arm was positioned in an AP/caudal view and then obliqued towards the patient's affected side until a definitive visualization of the targeted foramen with flattened vertebral endplates was demonstrated. The skin and subcutaneous tissues overlying the foramen were anesthetized. Using oblique and AP views, a 22-gauge spinal needle with a slight bend at the tip was advanced towards the inferior/posterior aspect of the foramen. An AP view was then used to advance the needle to approximately the center of the pillar or when patient response was noted. After negative aspiration to rule out vascular return, a non-ionic contrast was injected under live fluoroscopy confirming epidural spread through the foramen without vascular uptake. 1-2 cc of a mixture of 10mg/ml dexamethasone 1% lidocaine was injected into the epidural space. The needle was then removed, and hemostasis was achieved.

Disposition: Patient tolerated the procedure well without apparent complications. Patient was able to ambulate out of the facility in the same fashion they had entered. Discharge instructions were given.

Procedure name: Cervical Selective Nerve Root Block (SNRB)

Diagnosis:

Consent: The risks, benefits and anticipated outcomes of the procedure, the risks and benefits of the alternatives to the procedure, and the roles and tasks of the personnel involved, were discussed with the patient. The patient has given written informed consent to the procedure and agrees to proceed.

Anesthesia:

Attending physician:

Assisting physician:

Patient information:

Procedure detail: The patient was transported into the procedure room and was positioned supine on the fluoroscopy table. A time-out was performed per the usual clinical fashion. Monitors were placed and vital signs were observed throughout the procedure. The patient's head was turned away from the affected side. The patient's neck was prepped and draped in the usual sterile fashion. The C-arm was positioned in an AP/caudal view and then obliqued towards the patient affected side until a definitive visualization of the targeted foramen with flattened vertebral endplates demonstrated. The skin and subcutaneous tissues overlying the foramen was anesthetized. Using oblique and AP views, a 22-gauge spinal needle with a slight bend at the tip was advanced towards the inferior/posterior aspect of the foramen. An AP view was then used to advance the needle slightly inferior and lateral to the foramen or when patient response was noted. After negative aspiration to rule out vascular return, a non-ionic contrast was injected under live fluoroscopy demonstrating spread surrounding the dorsal root without vascular uptake. 1-2 cc of a mixture of 10mg/ml of dexamethasone and 1% lidocaine was then injected. The needle was then removed, and hemostasis was achieved.

Disposition: Patient tolerated the procedure well without apparent complications. Patient was able to ambulate out of the facility in the same fashion they had entered. Discharge instructions were given.

Procedure name: Cervical Intra-articular Facet Joint Injection

Diagnosis:

Consent: The risks, benefits and anticipated outcomes of the procedure, the risks and benefits of the alternatives to the procedure, and the roles and tasks of the personnel involved, were discussed with the patient. The patient has given written informed consent to the procedure and agrees to proceed.

Anesthesia:

Attending physician:

Assisting physician:

Patient information:

Procedure detail: The patient was transported into the procedure room and was positioned prone on the fluoroscopy table. A time-out was performed per the usual clinical fashion. Monitors were placed and vital signs were observed throughout the procedure. The patient's head was turned away from the affected side. The back of the patient's neck and upper back were prepped and draped in the usual sterile fashion. The C-arm was positioned in an AP view and then slightly contra-obliqued away from the patient's affected side so that the spinous process did not obscure the visualization of the facet joint. A caudal tilt was applied until the facet joint was demonstrated with clarity. The skin and subcutaneous tissues were anesthetized with 1% lidocaine. Without further adjustment of the C-arm, a 22-gauge spinal needle with a slight bend at the tip was advanced towards the pillar and after bone was reached, the curved tip of the needle was rotated to allow for advancement into the facet joint. After negative aspiration to rule out vascular return, contrast was injected under live fluoroscopy, a linear spread within the facet joint without vascular uptake was confirmed. 0.5 cc of a mixture of 10mg/ml dexamethasone and 1% lidocaine was injected into the epidural space. The needle was then removed, and hemostasis was achieved.

Disposition: The patient tolerated the procedure well without apparent complications. The patient was able to ambulate out of the facility in the same fashion they had entered. Discharge instructions were given.

Procedure name: Cervical Medial Branch Blocks (MBB)

Diagnosis:

Consent: The risks, benefits and anticipated outcomes of the procedure, the risks and benefits of the alternatives to the procedure, and the roles and tasks of the personnel involved, were discussed with the patient. The patient has given written informed consent to the procedure and agrees to proceed.

Anesthesia:

Attending physician:

Assisting physician:

Patient information:

Procedure detail: The patient was transported into the procedure room and was positioned prone on the fluoroscopy table. A time-out was performed per the usual clinical fashion. Monitors were placed and vital signs were observed throughout the procedure. The patient's head was turned away from the affected side. The back of the patient's neck and upper back was prepped and draped in the usual sterile fashion. The C-arm was positioned in an AP view and then slightly contra-obliqued away from the patient's affected side so that the spinous process did not obscure the visualization of the facet joint. A caudal tilt was applied until the facet joint was demonstrated with clarity. The skin was anesthetized with 1% lidocaine over cervical pillars, avoiding deep tissue. Without further adjustment of the C-arm, a 25-gauge spinal needle was advanced until bone was reached, and the tip of the needle was placed close to the concavity of the pillar. After negative aspiration to rule out vascular return, contrast was injected under live fluoroscopy demonstrating a curve spread around the pillar while confirming the absence vascular uptake. 1% lidocaine was injected. The needle was then removed, and hemostasis was achieved.

Disposition: The patient tolerated the procedure well without apparent complications. The patient was able to ambulate out of the facility in the same fashion they had entered. Discharge instructions were given.

Procedure name: Radiofrequency of Cervical Medial Branches

Diagnosis:

Consent: The risks, benefits and anticipated outcomes of the procedure, the risks and benefits of the alternatives to the procedure, and the roles and tasks of the personnel involved, were discussed with the patient. The patient has given written informed consent to the procedure and agrees to proceed.

Anesthesia:

Attending physician:

Assisting physician:

Patient information:

Procedure detail: The patient was transported into the procedure room and was positioned prone on the fluoroscopy table. A time-out was performed per the usual clinical fashion. Monitors were placed and vital signs were observed throughout the procedure. The patient's head was turned away from the affected side. The back of the patient's neck and upper back were prepped and draped in the usual sterile fashion. The C-arm was positioned in an AP view and then slightly obliqued towards the patient's affected side so that the spinous process did not obscure the visualization of the facet joint. A caudal tilt was applied until the facet joint was demonstrated with clarity. The skin was anesthetized with 1% lidocaine over cervical pillars, avoiding deep tissue. Without further adjustment of the C-arm, a radiofrequency needle was advanced until bone was reached, and the tip of the needle was placed close to the concavity of the pillar. Sensory testing was performed at 50 Hz with the patient confirming sensation at low voltage. Motor testing was then done at 2 Hz up to 2 millivolts while holding the distal extremity. Contractions of the multifidus muscle were noted during motor stimulation at all levels. Absence of muscle contraction in the extremity was confirmed at all levels. The electrodes were removed from the needles and 1% lidocaine was injected. The electrodes were then re-inserted into the needles and a fluoroscopic image was taken to confirm placement without alteration of the needle position. After 30 seconds to allow for local anesthetic to take effect, ablation was completed at 80ºC for 90 seconds. The electrode was removed, and 0.5% bupivacaine was injected. The needles were then removed, and hemostasis was achieved.

Medial branch	Sensory stimulation *(50Hz ~ 0.1-0.8V)*	Motor Stimulation without extremity contraction *(2Hz up to 2V)*
C4	<0.5	None
C5	<0.5	None
C6	<0.5	None
C7	<0.5	None

Disposition: The patient tolerated the procedure well without apparent complications. The patient was able to ambulate out of the facility in the same fashion they had entered. Discharge instructions were given.

Procedure name: Cervical Discography

Diagnosis:

Consent: The risks, benefits and anticipated outcomes of the procedure, the risks and benefits of the alternatives to the procedure, and the roles and tasks of the personnel involved, were discussed with the patient. The patient has given written informed consent to the procedure and agrees to proceed.

Anesthesia:

Attending physician:

Assisting physician:

Patient information:

Procedure detail: IV antibiotics were administered 30 minutes prior to the procedure. The patient was transported into the procedure room and positioned supine on the fluoroscopy table. A time-out was performed per the usual clinical fashion. Monitors were placed and vital signs were observed throughout the procedure. The patient's head was turned to the left. The C-arm was positioned in an AP/caudal view to flatten the endplates of the C6-7 level. The C-arm was then obliqued to the patient's right side until the superior articulating process was positioned posteriorly, allowing needle advancement parallel with the C-arm position. The skin and subcutaneous tissues overlying the disc space was anesthetized. AP, oblique and lateral views were used to position a 20-gauge, 1.5-inch introducer needle followed by a 25-gauge, 3-inch spinal needle with a slight bend at the tip was advanced via the introducer needle into the C6-7-disc nucleus. AP and lateral views were taken to confirm needle placement in the center of the disc. Using the same technique, needles were placed in the C5-6, C4-5, C3-4, and C2-3 disc respectively. Using a 1ml syringe, a mixture of contrast with an antibiotic was slowly injected into each disc while recording injection volume, disc appearance/findings, pain level and pain concordance. Based on pre-procedure imaging, normal appearing discs were tested first followed by suspected discs to influence accurateness of pain response.

During the testing stage, the patient was alert, oriented and unaware of the order the levels were being tested.

Level	Volume	Disc appearance/finding	Pain level	Concordant
C2-3	0.5ml	Normal appearance	***/10	Neg
C3-4	0.5ml	Normal appearance	***/10	Neg
C4-5	0.5ml	Normal appearance	***/10	Neg
C5-6	0.3ml	Anterior extravasation	***/10	Pos
C6-7	0.5ml	Normal appearance	***/10	Neg

After the levels were tested, 0.5 cc of 0.25% bupivacaine was injected into the discs. The needles were removed, hemostasis was achieved, and final images were taken.

Disposition: The patient tolerated the procedure well without apparent complications. The patient was able to ambulate out of the facility in the same fashion they had entered. Discharge instructions were given.

CHAPTER 3

THORACIC PROCEDURES

SAM SCIRE, R.T., (R)(CT), ARRT, CRT
AND K.C. MAASUMI, M.D., M.S.

List of procedures in this chapter:

- Interlaminar Epidural Steroid Injection
- Transforaminal Epidural Steroid Injection (TFESI)
- Medial Branch Block
- Medial Branch Radiofrequency Ablation
- Intercostal Nerve Injection

Procedure name: Interlaminar Epidural Steroid Injection

Diagnosis:

Consent: The risks, benefits and anticipated outcomes of the procedure, the risks and benefits of the alternatives to the procedure, and the roles and tasks of the personnel involved, were discussed with the patient. The patient has given written informed consent to the procedure and agrees to proceed.

Anesthesia:

Attending physician:

Assisting physician:

Patient information:

Procedure detail: The patient was transported into the procedure room and was positioned prone on the fluoroscopy table. A time-out was performed per the usual clinical fashion. Monitors were placed and vital signs were observed throughout the procedure. The patient's back was prepped and draped in a sterile manner. The C-arm was positioned in a true AP with a caudal tilt demonstrating an optimized view of the inter-laminar space. The skin and subcutaneous tissues overlying the inter-laminar space were anesthetized. Using AP and contralateral views, an 18-gauge Touhy needle with an attached loss of resistance syringe was advanced in a coaxial fashion until the ligamentum flavum was engaged and loss of resistance was obtained. After negative aspiration to rule out vascular return, contrast was injected under live fluoroscopy confirming epidural spread without vascular uptake. A mixture of 10 mg/ml of dexamethasone and 1% lidocaine was injected into the epidural space. The needle was then removed, and hemostasis was achieved.

Disposition: The patient tolerated the procedure well without apparent complications. The patient was able to ambulate out of the facility in the same fashion they had entered. Discharge instructions were given.

Procedure name: Transforaminal Epidural Steroid Injection (TFESI)

Diagnosis:

Consent: The risks, benefits and anticipated outcomes of the procedure, the risks and benefits of the alternatives to the procedure, and the roles and tasks of the personnel involved, were discussed with the patient. The patient has given written informed consent to the procedure and agrees to proceed.

Anesthesia:

Attending physician:

Assisting physician:

Patient information:

Procedure detail: The patient was transported into the procedure room and was positioned prone on the fluoroscopy table. A time-out was performed per the usual clinical fashion. Monitors were placed and vital signs were observed throughout the procedure. The patient's back was prepped and draped in a sterile manner. The skin and subcutaneous tissues overlying the foramen were anesthetized. Using AP and a slightly oblique contra-lateral view, a 22-gauge spinal needle with a slight bend at the tip was advanced towards the foramen and was positioned close to the foramen and/or when patient response was noted. The C-arm was then positioned in a lateral view to monitor the needle advancement into the posterior to mid foramen and/or when patient response was noted. After negative aspiration to rule out vascular return, contrast was injected under live fluoroscopy. Epidural spread through the foramen without vascular uptake was confirmed. A mixture of 10mg/ml of dexamethasone and 1% lidocaine was injected into the epidural space. The needle was then removed, and hemostasis was achieved. Fluoroscopic spot image(s) were taken to confirm the absence of a mediastinal pneumothorax.

Disposition: The patient tolerated the procedure well without apparent complications. The patient was able to ambulate out of the facility in the same fashion they had entered. Discharge instructions were given.

Procedure name: Medial Branch Block

Diagnosis:

Consent: The risks, benefits and anticipated outcomes of the procedure, the risks and benefits of the alternatives to the procedure, and the roles and tasks of the personnel involved, were discussed with the patient. The patient has given written informed consent to the procedure and agrees to proceed.

Anesthesia:

Attending physician:

Assisting physician:

Patient information:

Procedure detail: The patient was transported into the procedure room and was positioned prone on the fluoroscopy table. A time-out was performed per the usual clinical fashion. Monitors were placed and vital signs were observed throughout the procedure. The patient's back was prepped and draped in a sterile manner. Using a true AP view, a 25-gauge spinal needle with a slight bend at the tip, the needle was advanced to the superolateral edge of the transverse process until bone was reached. After negative aspiration to rule out vascular return, contrast was injected under live fluoroscopy confirming no vascular uptake and 1% lidocaine was injected. The needle was then removed, and hemostasis was achieved. Fluoroscopic spot image(s) were taken to confirm the absence of a pneumothorax.

Disposition: The patient tolerated the procedure well without apparent complications. The patient was able to ambulate out of the facility in the same fashion they had entered. Discharge instructions were given.

Procedure name: Medial Branch Radiofrequency Ablation

Diagnosis:

Consent: The risks, benefits and anticipated outcomes of the procedure, the risks and benefits of the alternatives to the procedure, and the roles and tasks of the personnel involved, were discussed with the patient. The patient has given written informed consent to the procedure and agrees to proceed.

Anesthesia:

Attending physician:

Assisting physician:

Patient information:

Procedure detail: The patient was transported into the procedure room and was positioned prone on the fluoroscopy table. A time-out was performed per the usual clinical fashion. Monitors were placed and vital signs were observed throughout the procedure. The patient's back was prepped and draped in a sterile manner. The skin was anesthetized using a small amount of 1% lidocaine to avoid interference during sensory and motor testing. Using a true AP view, a 22-gauge radiofrequency needle was placed at the superolateral edge of the transverse process until bone was reached. Sensory testing was performed at 50 Hz with the patient confirming sensation at low voltage. Motor testing was then done at 2 Hz up to 2 millivolts. Contractions of the multifidus muscle was noted during motor stimulation at all levels. The electrodes were removed from the needles and 1% lidocaine was injected. The electrodes were then re-inserted into the needles and a fluoroscopic image was taken to confirm placement without alteration of the needle position. After 30 seconds to allow for local anesthetic to take effect, ablation was done at 80ºC for 90 seconds. The electrodes were then removed, and a small amount of 0.5% bupivacaine was injected. The needles were then removed, and hemostasis was achieved. Fluoroscopic spot images were taken to confirm the absence of a mediastinal pneumothorax.

Medial branch	Sensory stimulation *(50Hz ~ 0.1-0.8V)*
T9	<0.5
T10	<0.5
T11	<0.5
T12	<0.5

Disposition: The patient tolerated the procedure well without apparent complications. The patient was able to ambulate out of the facility in the same fashion they had entered. Discharge instructions were given.

Procedure name: Intercostal Nerve Injection

Diagnosis:

Consent: The risks, benefits and anticipated outcomes of the procedure, the risks and benefits of the alternatives to the procedure, and the roles and tasks of the personnel involved, were discussed with the patient. The patient has given written informed consent to the procedure and agrees to proceed.

Anesthesia:

Attending physician:

Assisting physician:

Patient information:

Procedure detail: The patient was transported into the procedure room and was positioned prone on the fluoroscopy table. A time-out was performed per the usual clinical fashion. Monitors were placed and vital signs were observed throughout the procedure. The patient's back was prepped and draped in a sterile manner. Using a true AP view, the targeted rib was identified. The skin was anesthetized with 1% lidocaine slightly inferior to the rib. A 25-gauge needle with a slight bend at the tip was advanced to the inferior aspect of the rib until bone was reached. The needle was then carefully walked off the inferior aspect of the rib, advanced slightly and positioned underneath the rib into the costal grove. Contrast was injected showing a linear spread along the rib. A mixture of 10 mg/ml of dexamethasone and 1% lidocaine was injected. The needle was removed, and hemostasis was achieved. Fluoroscopic spot images were taken to confirm the absence of a pneumothorax.

Disposition: The patient tolerated the procedure well without apparent complications. The patient was able to ambulate out of the facility in the same fashion they had entered. Discharge instructions were given.

CHAPTER 4

LUMBAR PROCEDURES

SAM SCIRE, R.T., (R)(CT), ARRT, CRT
AND K.C. MAASUMI, M.D., M.S.

List of procedures in this chapter:

- Interlaminar Epidural Steroid Injection (LESI)
- Caudal Epidural Steroid Injection
- Caudal/Catheter Epidural Steroid Injection
- Transforaminal Epidural Steroid Injection (TFESI)
- Selective Nerve Root Block
- Sacral Foraminal Epidural Steroid Injection
- Interarticular Joint Injection
- Medial Branch Blocks
- Medial Branch Radiofrequency
- Lumbar Discography

Procedure name: Interlaminar Epidural Steroid Injection (LESI)

Diagnosis:

Consent: The risks, benefits and anticipated outcomes of the procedure, the risks and benefits of the alternatives to the procedure, and the roles and tasks of the personnel involved, were discussed with the patient. The patient has given written informed consent to the procedure and agrees to proceed.

Anesthesia:

Attending physician:

Assisting physician:

Patient information:

Procedure detail: The patient was transported into the procedure room and was positioned prone on the fluoroscopy table. A time-out was performed per the usual clinical fashion. Monitors were placed and vital signs were observed throughout the procedure. The patient's back was prepped and draped in a sterile manner. The C-arm was positioned in a true AP with a caudal tilt demonstrating an optimized view of the inter-laminar space. The skin and subcutaneous tissues overlying the inter-laminar space was anesthetized. Using AP and lateral views, an 18-gauge Touhy epidural needle with an attached loss of resistance syringe was advanced until the ligamentum flavum was engaged and loss of resistance was attained. After negative aspiration to rule out vascular return, contrast was injected under live fluoroscopy and epidural spread without vascular uptake was confirmed. A mixture of 10mg/ml of dexamethasone and 1% lidocaine was injected into the epidural space. The needle was then removed, and hemostasis was achieved.

Disposition: The patient tolerated the procedure well without apparent complications. The patient was able to ambulate out of the facility in the same fashion they had entered. Discharge instructions were given.

Procedure name: Caudal Epidural Steroid Injection

Diagnosis:

Consent: The risks, benefits and anticipated outcomes of the procedure, the risks and benefits of the alternatives to the procedure, and the roles and tasks of the personnel involved, were discussed with the patient. The patient has given written informed consent to the procedure and agrees to proceed.

Anesthesia:

Attending physician:

Assisting physician:

Patient information:

Procedure detail: The patient was transported into the procedure room and was positioned prone on the fluoroscopy table. A time-out was performed per the usual clinical fashion. Monitors were placed and vital signs were observed throughout the procedure. The patient's lower back and upper buttock were prepped and draped in a sterile manner. The C-arm was positioned in a lateral view demonstrating an optimized view of the sacral canal. The sacrococcygeal articulation was palpated and the overlying skin and subcutaneous tissues were anesthetized. Using a lateral view, an 18-gauge Touhy epidural needle was advanced into the sacral canal. After negative aspiration to rule out vascular return, contrast was injected under live fluoroscopy demonstrating spread within the sacral canal and without vascular uptake. A mixture of 10mg/ml of dexamethasone and 1% lidocaine was injected. The needle was then removed, and hemostasis was achieved.

Disposition: The patient tolerated the procedure well without apparent complications. The patient was able to ambulate out of the facility in the same fashion they had entered. Discharge instructions were given.

Procedure name: Caudal/Catheter Epidural Steroid Injection

Diagnosis:

Consent: The risks, benefits and anticipated outcomes of the procedure, the risks and benefits of the alternatives to the procedure, and the roles and tasks of the personnel involved, were discussed with the patient. The patient has given written informed consent to the procedure and agrees to proceed.

Anesthesia:

Attending physician:

Assisting physician:

Patient information:

Procedure detail: The patient was transported into the procedure room and was positioned prone on the fluoroscopy table. A time-out was performed per the usual clinical fashion. Monitors were placed and vital signs were observed throughout the procedure. The patient's lower back and upper buttock area were prepped and draped in a sterile manner. The C-arm was positioned in a lateral view demonstrating an optimized view of the sacral canal. The sacrococcygeal articulation was palpated and the overlying skin and subcutaneous tissues were anesthetized. Using a lateral view, an 18-gauge Touhy epidural needle was advanced into the sacral canal. After negative aspiration to rule out vascular return, a catheter was inserted and advanced through the needle to the L5 level. A true AP view was used to confirm placement at the L5 level. Contrast was injected under live fluoroscopy demonstrating spread within the epidural space and without vascular uptake. A mixture of 10mg/ml of dexamethasone and 1% lidocaine was injected. The catheter and needle were removed simultaneously, and hemostasis was achieved.

Disposition: The patient tolerated the procedure well without apparent complications. The patient was able to ambulate out of the facility in the same fashion they had entered. Discharge instructions were given.

Procedure name: Transforaminal Epidural Steroid Injection (TFESI)

Diagnosis:

Consent: The risks, benefits and anticipated outcomes of the procedure, the risks and benefits of the alternatives to the procedure, and the roles and tasks of the personnel involved, were discussed with the patient. The patient has given written informed consent to the procedure and agrees to proceed.

Anesthesia:

Attending physician:

Assisting physician:

Patient information:

Procedure detail: The patient was transported into the procedure room and was positioned prone on the fluoroscopy table. A time-out was performed per the usual clinical fashion. Monitors were placed and vital signs were observed throughout the procedure. The patient's back was prepped and draped in a sterile manner. The C-arm was positioned in a true AP view to identify the targeted level. The C-arm was then obliqued with a cephalic tilt demonstrating an enhanced view of the foramen. The skin and subcutaneous tissues overlying the foramen was anesthetized. A 22-gauge spinal needle with a slight bend at the tip was advanced towards the superior/posterior aspect of the foramen. The C-arm was then positioned in a true AP view and the needle was advanced to the 6 o'clock position just underneath the pedicle and/or when patient response was noted. After negative aspiration to rule out vascular return, contrast was injected under live fluoroscopy. Epidural spread through the foramen without vascular uptake was confirmed. A mixture of 10mg/ml of dexamethasone and 1% lidocaine was injected into the epidural space. The needle was then removed, and hemostasis was achieved.

Disposition: The patient tolerated the procedure well without apparent complications. The patient was able to ambulate out of the facility in the same fashion they had entered. Discharge instructions were given.

Procedure name: Selective Nerve Root Block

Diagnosis:

Consent: The risks, benefits and anticipated outcomes of the procedure, the risks and benefits of the alternatives to the procedure, and the roles and tasks of the personnel involved, were discussed with the patient. The patient has given written informed consent to the procedure and agrees to proceed.

Anesthesia:

Attending physician:

Assisting physician:

Patient information:

Procedure detail: The patient was transported into the procedure room and was positioned prone on the fluoroscopy table. A time-out was performed per the usual clinical fashion. Monitors were placed and vital signs were observed throughout the procedure. The patient's back was prepped and draped in a sterile manner. The C-arm was positioned in a true AP view to identify the targeted level. The C-arm was then obliqued with a cephalic tilt demonstrating an enhanced view of the foramen. The skin and subcutaneous tissues overlying the foramen was anesthetized. A 22-gauge spinal needle with a slight bend at the tip was advanced towards the mid/posterior and slightly inferior aspect of the foramen. The c-arm was then positioned in a true AP view and the needle was advanced slightly lateral to the 6 o'clock position underneath the pedicle or when patient response was noted. After negative aspiration to rule out vascular return, contrast was injected under live fluoroscopy. Contrast spread surrounding the dorsal root without vascular uptake was confirmed. A mixture of 10mg/ml of dexamethasone and 1% lidocaine was injected into the epidural space. The needle was then removed, and hemostasis was achieved.

Disposition: The patient tolerated the procedure well without apparent complications. The patient was able to ambulate out of the facility in the same fashion they had entered. Discharge instructions were given.

Procedure name: Sacral Foraminal Epidural Steroid Injection

Diagnosis:

Consent: The risks, benefits and anticipated outcomes of the procedure, the risks and benefits of the alternatives to the procedure, and the roles and tasks of the personnel involved, were discussed with the patient. The patient has given written informed consent to the procedure and agrees to proceed.

Anesthesia:

Attending physician:

Assisting physician:

Patient information:

Procedure detail: The patient was transported into the procedure room and was positioned prone on the fluoroscopy table. A time-out was performed per the usual clinical fashion. Monitors were placed and vital signs were observed throughout the procedure. The patient's lower back and upper buttock were prepped and draped in a sterile manner. The C-arm was positioned in a true AP view to identify the targeted level. The C-arm was then obliqued with a cephalic tilt demonstrating an enhanced view of the foramen. The skin and subcutaneous tissues overlying the foramen was anesthetized. A 22-gauge spinal needle with a slight bend at the tip was advanced towards the foramen. The C-arm was then positioned in a lateral view and the needle was further advanced into the sacral foramen or when patient response was noted. The C-arm was positioned back to an AP view. After negative aspiration to rule out vascular return, contrast was injected under live fluoroscopy. Epidural spread through the foramen without vascular uptake was confirmed. A mixture of 10mg/ml of dexamethasone and 1% lidocaine was injected into the epidural space. The needle was then removed, and hemostasis was achieved.

Disposition: The patient tolerated the procedure well without apparent complications. The patient was able to ambulate out of the facility in the same fashion they had entered. Discharge instructions were given.

Procedure name: Interarticular Facet Joint Injection

Diagnosis:

Consent: The risks, benefits and anticipated outcomes of the procedure, the risks and benefits of the alternatives to the procedure, and the roles and tasks of the personnel involved, were discussed with the patient. The patient has given written informed consent to the procedure and agrees to proceed.

Anesthesia:

Attending physician:

Assisting physician:

Patient information:

Procedure detail: The patient was transported into the procedure room and was positioned prone on the fluoroscopy table. A time-out was performed per the usual clinical fashion. Monitors were placed and vital signs were observed throughout the procedure. The patient's back was prepped and draped in a sterile manner. The C-arm was positioned in a true AP view to identify the targeted level. The C-arm was then obliqued demonstrating an enhanced view of the facet joint. The skin and subcutaneous tissues overlying the inferior aspect the facet joint was anesthetized. A 22-gauge spinal needle with a slight bend at the tip was advanced in a cephalic approach towards and then into the lower one third of the facet joint. After negative aspiration to rule out vascular return, contrast was injected under live fluoroscopy. A linear/oval spread within the facet joint without vascular uptake was confirmed. A mixture of 10mg/ml of dexamethasone and 1% lidocaine was injected into the facet joint. The needle was then removed, and hemostasis was achieved.

Disposition: The patient tolerated the procedure well without apparent complications. The patient was able to ambulate out of the facility in the same fashion they had entered. Discharge instructions were given.

Procedure name: Medial Branch Blocks

Diagnosis:

Consent: The risks, benefits and anticipated outcomes of the procedure, the risks and benefits of the alternatives to the procedure, and the roles and tasks of the personnel involved, were discussed with the patient. The patient has given written informed consent to the procedure and agrees to proceed.

Anesthesia:

Attending physician:

Assisting physician:

Patient information:

Procedure detail: The patient was transported into the procedure room and was positioned prone on the fluoroscopy table. A time-out was performed per the usual clinical fashion. Monitors were placed and vital signs were observed throughout the procedure. The patient's back and upper buttock were prepped and draped in a sterile manner. The C-arm was positioned in a true AP view to identify the targeted level(s). The C-arm was then obliqued demonstrating an enhanced view of the transverse and superior articulating processes. The skin overlying the junction of the transverse and superior articulating processes were anesthetized. A 22-gauge spinal needle with a slight bend at the tip was advanced to the superior articulating process/transverse process junction. Additional needles were placed in the same fashion at each level. Using a true AP view, a needle was also placed on the sacral ala slightly lateral to the superior articulating process of the sacrum. After negative aspiration to rule out vascular return, 1% lidocaine was injected through all needles. The needles were then removed, and hemostasis was achieved.

Disposition: The patient tolerated the procedure well without apparent complications. The patient was able to ambulate out of the facility in the same fashion they had entered. Discharge instructions were given.

Procedure name: Medial Branch Radiofrequency

Diagnosis:

Consent: The risks, benefits and anticipated outcomes of the procedure, the risks and benefits of the alternatives to the procedure, and the roles and tasks of the personnel involved, were discussed with the patient. The patient has given written informed consent to the procedure and agrees to proceed.

Anesthesia:

Attending physician:

Assisting physician:

Patient information:

Procedure detail: The patient was transported into the procedure room and was positioned prone on the fluoroscopy table. A time-out was performed per the usual clinical fashion. Monitors were placed and vital signs were observed throughout the procedure. The patient's back and upper buttock were prepped and draped in a sterile manner. Using a true AP view, the targeted level(s) were identified. The C-arm was obliqued with a significant caudal tilt. The skin just below the superior articulating process/transverse process junction at the intended vertebral level was anesthetized using a minimal amount of 1% lidocaine to avoid interference during sensory and motor testing. A 22-gauge radiofrequency needle was advanced parallel to the C-arm in both planes to the superior articulating process/transverse process junction lying more on the superior articulating process until bone was reached resulting in the needle placed parallel to the medial branch. An increased oblique and lateral views were used to confirm appropriate placement without the needle passing the superior articulating process thereby avoiding interaction with the motor nerve(s). The same technique was used to place RF needles at the other intended levels. Using a true AP view, a needle was also placed on the sacral ala slightly lateral to the superior articulating process of the sacrum. Sensory testing was performed at 50 Hz with the patient confirming sensation at low voltage. Motor testing was then done at 2 Hz up to 2 millivolts while holding the distal extremity. Contractions of the Multifidus was noted during motor stimulation. Absence of muscle contraction in the extremity was confirmed. The electrode was removed from the needle and 1% lidocaine was injected. The electrode was then re-inserted into the needle and a fluoroscopic image was taken to confirm placement without alteration of the needle position. After 30 seconds, to allow for local anesthetic to take effect, ablation was done at 80ºC for 90 seconds. The electrode was removed, and 0.5% bupivacaine was injected the needle(s) were then removed and hemostasis was achieved.

Medial branch	Sensory stimulation *(50Hz ~ 0.1-0.8V)*	Motor Stimulation without extremity contraction *(2Hz up to 2V)*
L3	< 0.5	None
L4	< 0.5	None
L5	< 0.5	None
Sacral Ala	< 0.5	None

Disposition: The patient tolerated the procedure well without apparent complications. The patient was able to ambulate out of the facility in the same fashion they had entered. Discharge instructions were given.

Procedure name: Lumbar Discography

Diagnosis:

Consent: The risks, benefits and anticipated outcomes of the procedure, the risks and benefits of the alternatives to the procedure, and the roles and tasks of the personnel involved, were discussed with the patient. The patient has given written informed consent to the procedure and agrees to proceed.

Anesthesia:

Attending physician:

Assisting physician:

Patient information:

Procedure detail: IV antibiotics were administered 30 minutes prior to the procedure. The patient was transported into the procedure room and positioned prone on the fluoroscopy table. A time-out was performed per the usual clinical fashion. Monitors were placed and vital signs were observed throughout the procedure. The patient's back and upper buttock were prepped and draped in a sterile manner. A cephalic tilt of the C-arm was positioned to flatten the endplates of the L5-S1 level. The C-arm was then obliqued to the patient's right side until the superior articulating process was positioned posteriorly to the center of the disc allowing needle advancement parallel with the C-arm position. The skin and subcutaneous tissues overlying the center of the disc were anesthetized. AP, oblique and lateral views were used to position a 20-gauge, 3-inch introducer needle followed by a 25-gauge, 6-inch spinal needle with a slight bend at the tip was advanced via the introducer needle into the intended disc nucleus. AP and lateral views were taken to confirm needle placement. Using the same technique, needles were placed in the intended discs respectively. A manometer was attached to the needles and a mixture of contrast with an antibiotic was slowly injected into each disc while recording opening, provocation and peak pressures, injection volume, disc appearance/findings, pain level and pain concordance. Based on pre-procedure imaging, normal appearing discs were tested first, followed by suspected discs to influence accurateness of pain response. During the testing stage, the patient was alert, oriented and unaware of the order the levels were being tested.

Pressures ---------------------

Level	Opening	Provocation	Concordant	Peak	Volume	Disc appearance/finding	Pain level	
L1-2	10		None	50	2.5ml	Normal appearance	***/10	Neg
L2-3	10		None	50	2.5ml	Normal appearance	***/10	Neg
L3-4	10		None	50	2.5ml	Normal appearance	***/10	Neg
L4-5	5		8	10	1.5ml	Anterior extravasation	***/10	Pos
L5-S1	10		None	50	2.5ml	Normal appearance	***/10	Neg

After the levels were tested, 0.5 ml of 0.25% bupivacaine was injected into the discs. The needles were removed, hemostasis was achieved, and final images were taken.

Disposition: The patient tolerated the procedure well without apparent complications. The patient was able to ambulate out of the facility in the same fashion they had entered. Discharge instructions were given.

CHAPTER 5

MINIMALLY INVASIVE SURGICAL PROCEDURES

K.C. MAASUMI, M.D., M.S.
AND SAM SCIRE, R.T., (R)(CT), ARRT, CRT

List of procedures in this chapter:

- Interlaminar Epidural Blood Patch Injection
- Kyphoplasty (Lumbar Spine)
- Vertebroplasty
- Spinal Cord Stimulator Trial
- Spinal Cord Stimulator Implant
- Intrathecal Injection
- Intrathecal Infusion Pump Implant
- Intrathecal Pump Catheter Dye Study
- Minimally Invasive Lumbar Decompression *(MILD)* procedure
- Interspinous Spacer
- Peripheral Nerve Stimulator Trial (Genicular Nerve)
- Peripheral Nerve Stimulator Implant (Genicular Nerve)
- Peripheral Nerve Stimulation Trial (Suprascapular Nerve)
- Peripheral Nerve Stimulation Implant (Suprascapular Nerve)

Procedure name: Interlaminar Epidural Blood Patch Injection

Diagnosis:

Consent: The risks, benefits and anticipated outcomes of the procedure, the risks and benefits of the alternatives to the procedure, and the roles and tasks of the personnel involved, were discussed with the patient. The patient has given written informed consent to the procedure and agrees to proceed.

Anesthesia:

Attending physician:

Assisting physician:

Patient information:

Procedure detail: The patient was transported into the procedure room and was positioned prone on the fluoroscopy table. A positioning aid was used to reduce lumbar lordosis. A time-out was performed per the usual clinical fashion. Monitors were placed and vital signs were observed throughout the procedure. The patient's back and right arm were prepped and draped in a sterile manner. An 18-gauge IV was placed in the right AC in the usual sterile fashion. The C-arm was positioned in a true AP with a caudal tilt demonstrating an optimized view of the L4-5 interlaminar space. The skin and subcutaneous tissues overlying the L4-5 interlaminar space were anesthetized. Using AP and lateral views, an 18-gauge Touhy epidural needle with an attached loss of resistance syringe was advanced until the ligamentum flavum was engaged and loss of resistance was attained. After negative aspiration to rule out vascular return, contrast was injected under live fluoroscopy and epidural spread without vascular uptake was confirmed. 10ml of blood was withdrawn from the patient's IV and was immediately injected into the epidural space. The needle was then removed, and hemostasis was achieved.

Disposition: The patient tolerated the procedure well without apparent complications. The patient was able to ambulate out of the facility in the same fashion they had entered. Discharge instructions were given.

Procedure name: Kyphoplasty (Lumbar Spine)

Diagnosis:

Consent: The risks, benefits and anticipated outcomes of the procedure, the risks and benefits of the alternatives to the procedure, and the roles and tasks of the personnel involved, were discussed with the patient. The patient has given written informed consent to the procedure and agrees to proceed.

Anesthesia:

Attending physician:

Assisting physician:

Patient information:

Procedure detail: The patient was transported into the procedure room and was positioned prone on the fluoroscopy table. A positioning aid was used to reduce lumbar lordosis. A time-out was performed per the usual clinical fashion. Monitors were placed and vital signs were observed throughout the procedure. The patient's back was prepped and draped in a sterile manner. The C-arm was positioned in a lateral position and a wig-wag adjustment was positioned to flatten the intended lumbar vertebral endplates to demonstrate a true lateral view. A true AP with a caudal tilt was made to flatten the endplates of the intended lumbar vertebral body. The C-arm was then obliqued towards the patient's left side until the pedicle was viewed parallel to the x-ray beam. Using a radiopaque marker, the entrance point was marked and the skin and subcutaneous tissues overlying the intended lumbar vertebral body's pedicle was anesthetized. A trocar was positioned parallel to the x-ray beam and advanced through the pedicle by carefully tapping the trocar with a mallet. After a slight loss of resistance, the C-arm was positioned to the lateral view showing the trocar path through the pedicle and then advanced with small taps with the mallet until the tip of the trocar was positioned close to the anterior wall of the vertebral body. The trocar was removed and the canula was retracted to the posterior third of the vertebral body. A balloon was inserted into the vertebral body with both balloon markers outside of the canula and within the vertebral body. The contrast filled balloon was inflated and viewed in both AP and lateral views showing a minimal lift of the superior endplate. The balloon was removed, and bone cement was slowly injected into the intended vertebral body while monitoring spot images in AP and lateral views. Cement spread throughout the vertebral body with augmented filling to the anterior-superior aspect of the vertebral body. Stabilization of the superior endplate and filling captivity within the vertebral body was noted. The trocar was inserted back into the canula and retracted into the pedicle for 30 seconds before removing simultaneously. Final AP and lateral views were taken, hemostasis was achieved, and bandages were applied.

Disposition: The patient tolerated the procedure well without apparent complications. The patient was able to ambulate out of the facility in the same fashion they had entered. Discharge instructions were given.

Procedure name: Vertebroplasty

Diagnosis:

Consent: The risks, benefits and anticipated outcomes of the procedure, the risks and benefits of the alternatives to the procedure, and the roles and tasks of the personnel involved, were discussed with the patient. The patient has given written informed consent to the procedure and agrees to proceed.

Anesthesia:

Attending physician:

Assisting physician:

Patient information:

Procedure detail: The patient was transported into the procedure room and was positioned prone on the fluoroscopy table. A positioning aid was used to reduce lumbar lordosis. A time-out was performed per the usual clinical fashion. Monitors were placed and vital signs were observed throughout the procedure. The patient's back was prepped and draped in a sterile manner. The C-arm was positioned in a lateral position and a wig-wag adjustment was positioned to flatten the L1 endplates to demonstrate a true lateral view. A true AP with a caudal tilt was made to flatten the endplates of L1. The C-arm was then obliqued towards the patient's left side until the pedicle was viewed parallel to the x-ray beam. Using a radiopaque marker, the entrance point was marked and the skin and subcutaneous tissues overlying left L1 pedicle was anesthetized. A trocar was positioned parallel to the x-ray beam and advanced through the pedicle by carefully tapping the trocar with a mallet. After a slight loss of resistance, the lateral view was viewed and the trocar path through the pedicle was confirmed with the tip advanced close to the anterior wall of the vertebral body. The trocar was removed and the canula was retracted to the posterior third of the vertebral body. A manual drill was inserted through the canula into the vertebral body and under live fluoroscopy was used to extract bone. Cement was slowly injected into the L1 vertebral body while taking frequent spot images in the lateral view. Cement spread throughout the vertebral body bilaterally with increased spread to the anterior-superior aspect of the vertebral body and was confined within the vertebral body. The trocar was inserted back into the tube and retracted into the pedicle for 30 seconds before removing the tube and stylet simultaneously. Final AP and lateral views were taken, hemostasis was achieved, and bandages were applied.

Disposition: The patient tolerated the procedure well without apparent complications. The patient was able to ambulate out of the facility in the same fashion they had entered. Discharge instructions were given.

Procedure name: Spinal Cord Stimulator Trial

Diagnosis:

Consent: The risks, benefits and anticipated outcomes of the procedure, the risks and benefits of the alternatives to the procedure, and the roles and tasks of the personnel involved, were discussed with the patient. The patient has given written informed consent to the procedure and agrees to proceed.

Anesthesia:

Attending physician:

Assisting physician:

Patient information:

Procedure detail: The patient was transported into the procedure room and positioned prone on the fluoroscopy table with a positioning aid to reduce lumbar lordosis. A time-out was performed per the usual clinical fashion. Monitors were placed and vital signs were observed throughout the procedure. The patient's mid-lower back was prepped and draped in a sterile manner. The C-arm was positioned in a lateral position and a wig-wag adjustment was positioned to flatten the Thoraco-lumbar endplates to demonstrate a true lateral view. A true AP with a caudal tilt demonstrating an optimized view of the T12-L1 interlaminar space. The overlying skin and subcutaneous tissues just medial/inferior to the right L2 pedicle were anesthetized. Using a lateral-medial approach, an 18-gauge Touhy needle with an attached loss of resistance syringe was advanced until the ligamentum flavum was engaged and loss of resistance was attained. After negative aspiration to rule out vascular return, an eight-lead stimulator electrode was advanced into the epidural space. While checking true AP and lateral views, the electrode was positioned with the tip of the electrode at mid T7 and the eighth electrode at mid T9. Prior to testing the patient was assessed for alertness, orientation, and the ability to proceed to the testing phase. The patient confirmed the masking of pain during stimulation. The needle was removed, and spot images were taken to confirm placement of the electrode. The same technique was repeated on the left side for bilateral stimulation. The wires were connected to the generator and a sterile dressing was applied. The patient was then transferred to post procedure recovery where further testing was performed by the product representative.

Disposition: The patient tolerated the procedure well without apparent complications. The patient was able to ambulate out of the facility in the same fashion they had entered. Discharge instructions were given.

Procedure name: Spinal Cord Stimulator Implant

Diagnosis:

Consent: The risks, benefits and anticipated outcomes of the procedure, the risks and benefits of the alternatives to the procedure, and the roles and tasks of the personnel involved, were discussed with the patient. The patient has given written informed consent to the procedure and agrees to proceed.

Anesthesia:

Attending physician:

Assisting physician:

Patient information:

Procedure detail: The patient was transported into the procedure room and positioned prone on the fluoroscopy table with a positioning aid to reduce lumbar lordosis. A time-out was performed per the usual clinical fashion. Monitors were placed and vital signs were observed throughout the procedure. The patient's mid-lower back was prepped and draped in a sterile manner. The C-arm was positioned in a lateral position and a wig-wag adjustment was positioned to flatten the Thoraco-lumbar endplates to demonstrate a true lateral view. A true AP with a caudal tilt was applied to open the T12-L1 interlaminar space. The overlying skin and subcutaneous tissues just medial/inferior to the right L2 pedicle were anesthetized. Using a lateral-medial approach, an 18-gauge Touhy needle with an attached loss of resistance syringe was advanced until the ligamentum flavum was engaged and loss of resistance was attained. After negative aspiration to rule out vascular return, an eight-lead stimulator electrode was advanced into the epidural space. While checking true AP and lateral views, the electrode was positioned with the tip of the electrode at mid T7 and the eighth electrode at mid T9. Prior to testing the patient was assessed for alertness, orientation, and the ability to proceed to the testing phase. The patient confirmed the masking of pain during stimulation. The needle was removed, and spot images were taken to confirm placement of the electrode. The same technique was repeated on the left side for bilateral stimulation. Both electrodes were sutured to the facia using 4-0 suture Prolene (non-absorbable, sterile suture that is made of isotactic crystalline steroisomer of polypropylene).

A surgical pocket was made in the left upper buttock. Cauterization was used as necessary to control bleeding. Lidocaine with epinephrine was injected into subcutaneous tissues to anesthetize the path of the tunnel. A tunnel was made from the surgical pocket to the electrode entrance site. The electrodes were placed through the tunnel into the surgical pocket and then attached to the generator. The pocket was rinsed with antibiotic irrigation to reduce the risk of infection. A powder antibiotic was also placed into the pocket as well. The generator was then placed into the surgical pocket and then the pocket was closed using 3-0 Monocryl and 4-0 Vicryl (absorbable, synthetic, suture). Dermabond was applied to the skin followed by a sterile dressing. The patient was then transferred to post procedure recovery where further testing was performed by the product representative.

Disposition: The patient tolerated the procedure well without apparent complications. The patient was able to ambulate out of the facility in the same fashion they had entered. Discharge instructions were given.

Procedure name: Intrathecal Injection

Diagnosis:

Consent: The risks, benefits and anticipated outcomes of the procedure, the risks and benefits of the alternatives to the procedure, and the roles and tasks of the personnel involved, were discussed with the patient. The patient has given written informed consent to the procedure and agrees to proceed.

Anesthesia:

Attending physician:

Assisting physician:

Patient information:

Procedure detail: The patient was transported into the procedure room and positioned prone on the fluoroscopy table with a positioning aid to reduce lumbar lordosis. A time-out was performed per the usual clinical fashion. Monitors were placed and vital signs were observed throughout the procedure. The patient's lower back was prepped and draped in a sterile manner. The C-arm was positioned in an AP position with adjustments to define the L2-3 interlaminar space. A 22-gauge spinal needle was advanced until the return of CSF was confirmed. Contrast was injected. AP and lateral views demonstrated a striated appearance with contrast retainment in the subarachnoid space. 100 mcg of morphine was injected, the needle was then removed, and hemostasis was achieved.

Disposition: The patient tolerated the procedure well without apparent complications. The patient was able to ambulate out of the facility in the same fashion they had entered. Discharge instructions were given.

Procedure name: Intrathecal Infusion Pump Implant

Diagnosis:

Consent: The risks, benefits and anticipated outcomes of the procedure, the risks and benefits of the alternatives to the procedure, and the roles and tasks of the personnel involved, were discussed with the patient. The patient has given written informed consent to the procedure and agrees to proceed.

Anesthesia:

Attending physician:

Assisting physician:

Patient information:

Procedure detail: The patient was transported into the procedure room and positioned left side down on the fluoroscopy table. A time-out was performed per the usual clinical fashion. Monitors were placed and vital signs were observed throughout the procedure. The patient's mid-lower back and abdomen were prepped and draped in a sterile manner. The C-arm was positioned in a lateral position and a wig-wag adjustment was positioned to demonstrate a cross-table AP view at L2-3. The overlying skin and subcutaneous tissues were anesthetized with 1% lidocaine. A posterior midline incision overlying L2-3 was made from the skin to the supraspinous fascia. Electrocautery was used to control bleeding and maintain hemostasis. A 16-gauge Touhy spinal needle is advanced through the incision into the subarachnoid space confirmed with the return of CSF. A catheter was advanced within the intrathecal space up to T10. A lateral view was then checked to confirm appropriate placement. The Touhy needle was removed, and the provided anchor was placed over the catheter and was sutured to the supraspinous fascia using 3-0 silk. The skin and subcutaneous tissues in the RLQ indicating the pocket opening was anesthetized with 1% lidocaine. A horizontal linear incision slightly wider than the infusion pump was made in the RLQ of the abdomen. Electrocautery was used to control bleeding and maintain hemostasis. A pocket slightly larger than the pump was formed. Using a tunneling device, a tunnel was made from the supraspinous incision to the pocket. The catheter was advanced through the tunnel device, trimmed and attached to the infusion pump leaving some slack at both ends of the catheter. The pocket was irrigated with an antibiotic rinse and there was no residual bleeding. A powder antibiotic was placed in the pocket followed by the placement of the pump. The subcutaneous tissue and skin of both incisions were closed with 3-0 Monocryl and 2-0 Vicryl respectively. Sterile dressing was then applied. The patient was then transferred to post procedure recovery where further testing was performed by the product representative.

Disposition: The patient tolerated the procedure well without apparent complications. The patient was able to ambulate out of the facility in the same fashion they had entered. Discharge instructions were given.

Procedure name: Intrathecal Pump Catheter Dye Study

Diagnosis:

Consent: The risks, benefits and anticipated outcomes of the procedure, the risks and benefits of the alternatives to the procedure, and the roles and tasks of the personnel involved, were discussed with the patient. The patient has given written informed consent to the procedure and agrees to proceed.

Anesthesia:

Attending physician:

Assisting physician:

Patient information:

Procedure detail: The patient was transported into the procedure room and was positioned supine on the fluoroscopy table. A time-out was performed per the usual clinical fashion. Monitors were placed and vital signs were observed throughout the procedure. A representative was present to assist with the infusion pump operation and the pump was turned off. Initial fluoroscopic images were taken. The catheter appeared to be intact without any kinks, displacement and/or catheter/pump connection issues. The patient's abdomen was prepped and draped in a sterile manner. The C-arm was positioned in an AP position and angular adjustments were made so that the catheter port was well visualized. The overlying skin and subcutaneous tissues were anesthetized. The catheter port was engaged with a needle provided by the representative. Negative aspiration was applied to remove all medication from the catheter. Contrast dye was introduced and injected through the catheter under live fluoroscopy. Filling defects in the catheter was ruled out. Negative aspiration was again applied to remove as much contrast dye as possible and the pump was programed to refill the catheter with medication and continue infusion as programmed. The needle was removed, hemostasis was achieved, and an adhesive bandage was applied.

Disposition: The patient tolerated the procedure well without apparent complications. The patient was able to ambulate out of the facility in the same fashion they had entered. Discharge instructions were given.

Procedure name: Minimally Invasive Lumbar Decompression *(MILD)* Procedure

Diagnosis:

Consent: The risks, benefits and anticipated outcomes of the procedure, the risks and benefits of the alternatives to the procedure, and the roles and tasks of the personnel involved, were discussed with the patient. The patient has given written informed consent to the procedure and agrees to proceed.

Anesthesia:

Attending physician:

Assisting physician:

Patient information:

Procedure detail: An antibiotic was given 30 minutes prior to the start of the procedure. The patient was transported into the procedure room and was positioned prone on the fluoroscopy table with a positioning aid to reduce lumbar lordosis. A time-out was performed per the usual clinical fashion. Monitors were placed and vital signs were observed throughout the procedure. The patient's mid-lower back was prepped and draped in a sterile manner. The C-arm was positioned in a true AP and the L3-4 interlaminar space was identified. The overlying skin and subcutaneous tissues were anesthetized with 1% lidocaine. An 18-gauge Touhy needle with an attached loss of resistance syringe was advanced until the ligamentum flavum was engaged and loss of resistance was attained. After negative aspiration to rule out vascular return, contrast was injected demonstrating a linear spread with stenotic appearance and resistance of contrast spread at the L3-4 level. The Touhy needle remained in the epidural space during the procedure to allow for additional contrast to be injected as needed to ensure visualization of the epidural space. The C-arm was then obliqued towards the patient's left side. The skin and subcutaneous tissue just inferior to the lamina were anesthetized with 1% lidocaine. A 22-gauge spinal needle was advanced to the L4 lamina with a cephalic approach to the lateral edge of the spinous process of the inferior lamina, and 1% lidocaine was used to anesthetize the track. A contralateral oblique view was used to confirm depth. The provided trocar/cannula system was advanced to the L4 lamina. Depth placement is confirmed with a contralateral oblique view and contact. The MILD portal stabilizer was then secured on the patient. The trocar was removed, and the depth guide was placed onto the top of the portal. Removal of small amounts of bone of the lamina was achieved using the provided bone rongeur followed by the tissue sculptor to remove small sections of Ligamentum Flavum. Multiple passes were performed with the bone rongeur and tissue sculptor until a micro-laminectomy was achieved and tissue debulking was accomplished. Contrast was injected though the Touhy needle which subsequently demonstrated increased flow beyond the pre-procedure spot of resistance. The Touhy needle and MILD system was removed. Reinforced adhesive skin closures like Steri-strips followed by a sterile bandage were used to close the incision wound.

Disposition: The patient tolerated the procedure well without apparent complications. The patient was able to ambulate out of the facility in the same fashion they had entered. Discharge instructions were given.

Procedure name: Interspinous Spacer

Diagnosis:

Consent: The risks, benefits and anticipated outcomes of the procedure, the risks and benefits of the alternatives to the procedure, and the roles and tasks of the personnel involved, were discussed with the patient. The patient has given written informed consent to the procedure and agrees to proceed.

Anesthesia:

Attending physician:

Assisting physician:

Patient information:

Procedure detail: The patient was transported into the procedure room and was positioned prone on the fluoroscopy table. A positioning aid was used to reduce lumbar lordosis. A time-out was performed per the usual clinical fashion. Monitors were placed and vital signs were observed throughout the procedure. The patient's lower back was prepped and draped in a sterile manner. The C-arm was positioned in a lateral position and a wig-wag adjustment was made to flatten the L3-4 endplates. The C-arm was then positioned in a true AP with a caudal tilt to separate the L3 and L4 spinous processes. The overlying skin and subcutaneous tissues between the L3 and L4 spinous processes were anesthetized. A small entrance incision was made mid-line between the L3 and L4 spinous process. A blunt dilator was introduced and advanced parallel to the spinous processes. The C-arm was then positioned to the lateral view to monitor depth while further advancing the dilator until the tip reached the dorsal aspect of the facet shadow. AP and lateral views were taken to confirm midline and depth placement. A canula was then inserted and advanced over the dilator until it was firmly seated between the L3 and L4 spinous processes and approximately 10mm dorsal to the spinolaminar junction. AP and lateral views were again taken to confirm midline and depth placement. The dilator was removed followed by the insertion of the reamer to remove tissue within the canula. AP and lateral views were taken to confirm positioning and orientation. The gauge measuring device was positioned through the canula actuated until resistance was attained. A 12-gauge implant was selected. The gauge was removed, and the implant deployment device was inserted through the canula. AP and lateral views were again taken to confirm positioning, orientation, and alignment. Using intermittent fluoroscopy, the deployment device was adjusted posteriorly as the implant was being deployed. Soft tapping on the deployment device was applied to ensure firm seating and the implant body was placed at the spinolaminar junction. The implant was then detached, and all instruments were removed. Final AP and lateral spot images were obtained. The incision was irrigated with an antibiotic rinse and closed with a 3-0 Vicryl. Steri-strips and sterile bandage were applied.

Disposition: The patient tolerated the procedure well without apparent complications. The patient was able to ambulate out of the facility in the same fashion they had entered. Discharge instructions were given.

Procedure name: Peripheral Nerve Stimulator Trial (Genicular Nerve)

Diagnosis:

Consent: The risks, benefits and anticipated outcomes of the procedure, the risks and benefits of the alternatives to the procedure, and the roles and tasks of the personnel involved, were discussed with the patient. The patient has given written informed consent to the procedure and agrees to proceed.

Anesthesia:

Attending physician:

Assisting physician:

Patient information:

Procedure detail: Antibiotics was infused 30 minutes prior to the start of the procedure. The patient was brought into the procedure room and positioned supine on the fluoroscopy table with the affected knee flexed about 20 degrees supported with a pillow or foam. The affected knee was cleaned and draped in a sterile fashion. An anterior-posterior fluoroscopic view of the affected tibiofemoral joint was obtained with an open tibiofemoral joint space and equal width interspaces on both sides. The junctions connecting the tibial shaft to the inferior medial epicondyle was marked. Skin and soft tissues were anesthetized with 1 mL 1% lidocaine. Under fluoroscopic guidance, a 25-gauge 3.5-inch spinal needles with curved tip was advanced percutaneously towards areas connecting the shaft to the epicondyle, abutting the bone. A lateral fluoroscopic view was obtained, and needles were adjusted at the midline of the diaphysis and advanced to approximately 50-75% of the depth of femur.

Using a 15 blade, a small incision was made at the appropriate location in such a way that the two receiver points remain outside of the body. Then in lateral view, an introducer was inserted and carefully advance under fluoroscopic guidance until the tip of it reached the flare of the tibia. The stylet was then removed. The lead was inserted to the proper location with the tip at the tibial flare within 1-2 cm away from the tibial bone. The stylet of the lead was removed, and the antenna was inserted without kinking. Then the space of the lead farther from the second receiver point was tied securely.

Imaging confirmed that the lead did not move. At the incision location where the lead is coming out, Steri-strips were used to secure the lead in a chevron pattern, and Transparent film dressing was used on top of it to secure it. Representative from the vendor tested the device.

Disposition: The patient tolerated the procedure well without apparent complications. The patient was able to ambulate out of the facility in the same fashion they had entered. Discharge instructions were given.

Procedure name: Peripheral Nerve Stimulator Implant (Genicular Nerve)

Diagnosis:

Consent: The risks, benefits and anticipated outcomes of the procedure, the risks and benefits of the alternatives to the procedure, and the roles and tasks of the personnel involved, were discussed with the patient. The patient has given written informed consent to the procedure and agrees to proceed.

Anesthesia:

Attending physician:

Assisting physician:

Patient information:

Procedure detail: The patient received 1-gram cefazolin IV. She was brought into the procedure room and positioned supine on the fluoroscopy table with the left knee flexed about 20 degrees supported with a foam. The affected right knee was placed in neutral position and cleaned and draped in a sterile fashion from the bottom of the foot to middle of the right thigh. An anterior-posterior fluoroscopic view of the affected tibiofemoral joint was obtained with equal width interspaces on both sides. The junctions connecting the tibial shaft to the inferior medial epicondyle was marked. Skin and soft tissues were anesthetized with 1 mL 1% lidocaine prior to needle insertion. Under fluoroscopic guidance, a 25-gauge 3.5-inch spinal needles was advanced percutaneously towards area connecting the shaft to the epicondyle, abutting the bone. A lateral fluoroscopic view was obtained, and needles were adjusted at the midline of the diaphysis and advanced to approximately 50-75% of the depth of femur.

Using a 15 blade, a small vertical incision, 0.5 cm in length was made at the appropriate location in such a way that the two receiver points remain outside of the body. Then in lateral view, an introducer was inserted and carefully advance under fluoroscopic guidance until the tip of it reached the flare of the tibia. The stylet was then removed. The lead was inserted to the proper location with the tip at the tibial flare within 1-2 cm away from the tibial bone. The stylet of the lead was removed, and the antenna was inserted without kinking. Another 2 cm vertical incision was made inferior to the initial incision in such a way that the lead space between the two antennas would be tunneled under the skin. The same yellow introducer was used to tunnel the lead. The end of the lead was tied tight with one knot. A coil was made about 1-2 cm in diameter. The two sides of the circular coil was tied with non-absorbable suture. A suture was placed in the fascia. The coil was secured in place with the end of the probe facing down. The incision inferiorly was closed in two layers with two 4-0 absorbable suture and then with 2-0 absorbable suture on the skin. The superior incision was closed in one layer with 2-0 absorbable suture. Reinforced adhesive skin closures were applied to both incisions and a Transparent film dressing was applied on top. The patient was transported to the post op room. She tolerated the procedure well. Representative from the vendor tested the device by stimulation.

Disposition: The patient tolerated the procedure well without apparent complications. Discharge instructions were given.

Procedure name: Peripheral Nerve Stimulation Trial (Suprascapular Nerve)

Diagnosis:

Consent: The risks, benefits and anticipated outcomes of the procedure, the risks and benefits of the alternatives to the procedure, and the roles and tasks of the personnel involved, were discussed with the patient. The patient has given written informed consent to the procedure and agrees to proceed.

Anesthesia:

Attending physician:

Assisting physician:

Patient information:

Procedure detail: Patient was brought into the procedure room and positioned prone on the fluoroscopy table with arm tucked on the side. The affected shoulder was cleaned and draped in a sterile fashion. An anterior-posterior fluoroscopic view of the affected shoulder joint was obtained. The coracoid process and the suprascapular notch as well as scapular spine were identified.

The lead was placed on the skin to ensure proper location of the incision. The location was anesthetized. A 15 blade was used to create a small incision 1 cm distal to lead marker for insertion of the introducer. The introducer was guided via fluoroscopy from medial to lateral location, staying superficial first and then once over the scapular spine, deep into the tissue close to the suprascapular notch. Once in the proper location, the stimulator lead was guided through the introducer. The guide was removed with the lead in proper location. A chevron Steri-strip was used to secure the lead. Sterile Transparent film dressing was place over the lead. The end of the lead after the antenna was tied and cut. Lastly imaging was obtained to ensure the lead is in the proper place.

Disposition: The patient tolerated the procedure well without apparent complications. Discharge instructions were given.

Procedure name: Peripheral Nerve Stimulation Implant (Suprascapular Nerve)

Diagnosis:

Consent: The risks, benefits and anticipated outcomes of the procedure, the risks and benefits of the alternatives to the procedure, and the roles and tasks of the personnel involved, were discussed with the patient. The patient has given written informed consent to the procedure and agrees to proceed.

Anesthesia:

Attending physician:

Assisting physician:

Patient information:

Procedure detail: The patient was brought into the procedure room and positioned prone on the fluoroscopy table with arm tucked on the side. The affected shoulder was cleaned and draped in a sterile fashion. Antimicrobial drape was used over the affected area. An anterior-posterior fluoroscopic view of the affected shoulder joint was obtained. The coracoid process and the suprascapular notch as well as scapular spine were identified by having a 5 degree cephalad tilt.

The lead was placed on the skin to ensure proper location of the incision. The location was anesthetized. A 15 blade was used to create a small incision 1 cm distal to lead marker for insertion of the introducer. The introducer was guided via fluoroscopy from medial to lateral location, staying superficial first and then once over the scapular spine, deep into the tissue close to the suprascapular notch. Once in the proper location, the stimulator lead was guided through the introducer. The guide was removed with the lead in proper location. Then a 90-degree turn was made placing the remainder of the lead vertically down lateral to the spinous process. An incision was made below the marker on the lead and the lead was tunneled. The end of the lead was tied, and a "pretzel" tie was made additionally to help anchoring. The bottom of the lead with the ties was anchored to the fascia and tucked into a pocket. The tie itself was also tied via non absorbable sutures. The two incisions were sutured with non-absorbable sutures. Lastly imaging was obtained to ensure the lead is in the proper place.

Disposition: The patient tolerated the procedure well without apparent complications. Discharge instructions were given.

CHAPTER 6

JOINT INJECTIONS

K.C. MAASUMI, M.D., M.S.

Procedure in this chapter:

- Glenohumeral Joint Steroid Injection
- Acromioclavicular Joint Injection
- Sacroiliac Joint Injection
- Intra-articular Joint Injection
- Genicular Nerve Block
- Genicular Nerve Radiofrequency Ablation
- Femoral and obturator Nerve Block
- Intra-articular Hip Injection

Procedure name: Glenohumeral Joint Steroid Injection

Diagnosis:

Consent: The risks, benefits and anticipated outcomes of the procedure, the risks and benefits of the alternatives to the procedure, and the roles and tasks of the personnel to be involved, were discussed with the patient. The patient has given written informed consent to the procedure and agrees to proceed.

Anesthesia:

Attending physician:

Assisting physician:

Patient information:

Procedure detail: The patient was brought into the procedure room and positioned seated with shoulders exposed. The area was marked and then prepped in the usual sterile fashion. A linear ultrasound probe with sterile covering was used to view the subacromial bursa with the transducer oriented in the coronal/scapular plane and positioned just over the tip of the acromion. The bursa was seen as a thin anechoic fluid layer immediately above the tendon. The area of interest was anesthetized locally. Then a 21-gauge, 10 cm hyperechoic ultrasound needle was advanced under ultrasound guidance to reach the joint space. 2-3 cc of medication consisting of 10m/ml dexamethasone and 1% lidocaine was injected into the joint space.

Disposition: The patient tolerated the procedure well without apparent complications. Patient was able to ambulate out of the facility in the same fashion they had entered. Discharge instructions were given.

Procedure name: Acromioclavicular Joint Injection

Diagnosis:

Consent: The risks, benefits and anticipated outcomes of the procedure, the risks and benefits of the alternatives to the procedure, and the roles and tasks of the personnel to be involved, were discussed with the patient. The patient has given written informed consent to the procedure and agrees to proceed

Anesthesia:

Attending physician:

Assisting physician:

Patient information:

Procedure detail: The patient was brought into the procedure room and positioned seated. The affected shoulder was cleaned and prepped in a sterile fashion. A linear ultrasound probe was used to image the acromioclavicular joint with transducer oriented in the coronal plane and positioned just over the tip of the acromion distal to the clavicle. Using a 27-gauge 1.5-inch needle, 1 mL of 1% lidocaine was used as local anesthetic. 1 cc of a solution consisting of 10mg/ml dexamethasone and 1% lidocaine was injected into the joint. After injection, the joint was passively moved through the full range of motion. The patient tolerated the procedure well.

Disposition: The patient tolerated the procedure well without apparent complications. The patient was able to ambulate out of the facility in the same fashion they had entered. Discharge instructions were given.

Procedure name: Sacroiliac Joint Injection

Diagnosis:

Consent: The risks, benefits and anticipated outcomes of the procedure, the risks and benefits of the alternatives to the procedure, and the roles and tasks of the personnel to be involved, were discussed with the patient. The patient has given written informed consent to the procedure and agrees to proceed.

Anesthesia:

Attending physician:

Assisting physician:

Patient information:

Procedure detail: The patient was brought into the procedure room and placed prone on the fluoroscopy table. Standard monitors were placed, and vital signs were observed throughout the procedure. The area of the low back and sacrum was prepped and draped in a sterile manner. The affected sacroiliac joint was identified and marked under AP fluoroscopy. The fluoroscopic beam was then obliqued to align the anterior and posterior margins of sacroiliac joint. The inferior margin of the joint was identified and marked. The skin and subcutaneous tissues in these areas were anesthetized with 1% lidocaine. A 23-gauge, 3.5-inch spinal needle was advanced toward the targeted point under fluoroscopic guidance. Once the targeted point was reached and the joint space entered, lateral fluoroscopy was used to confirm advancement of the needle tip beyond the posterior sacral plate. Once negative aspiration was confirmed, 2-3 cc solution consisting of 10mg/ml dexamethasone and 1% lidocaine was injected. The needle was restyletted and removed with the tip intact.

Disposition: The patient tolerated the procedure well without apparent complications. The patient was able to ambulate out of the facility in the same fashion they had entered. Discharge instructions were given.

Procedure name: Intra-articular Knee Joint Injection

Diagnosis:

Consent: The risks, benefits and anticipated outcomes of the procedure, the risks and benefits of the alternatives to the procedure, and the roles and tasks of the personnel to be involved, were discussed with the patient. The patient has given written informed consent to the procedure and agrees to proceed.

Anesthesia:

Attending physician:

Assisting physician:

Patient information:

Procedure detail: The patient was brought into the procedure room and positioned prone on the table with the affected knee flexed at 20 degrees. The affected knee was prepped and draped in the sterile fashion. A linear high-resolution transducer with sterile probe cover was placed longitudinally parallel to the tendon of quadriceps femoris muscle. The distal femur, the superior pole of the patella, suprapatellar fat pad and the suprapatellar recess were visualized. The transducer was then rotated to the axial plane, and tendon of quadriceps femoris, suprapatellar fat pad, and the suprapatellar bursa were identified. The skin and subcutaneous tissues overlying this were anesthetized with 1% lidocaine using a 27-gauge 1.25-inch needle. Following the same needle trajectory, a 21gauge 10cm hyperechoic ultrasound needle was advanced under direct ultrasound visualization to the joint. 2-3 cc of solution consisting of 10mg/ml dexamethasone and 1% lidocaine was injected into the joint space while observing the suprapatellar pouch filling in real time under ultrasound. Please note that Hyaluronic Acid can be injected in the same fashion. The needle was restyletted and removed with the tip intact. Hemostasis was easily achieved.

The same procedure can be done under fluoroscopy.

An anterior-posterior view of the affected knee is obtained with the patella in center and joint space maximized. Under direct fluoroscopic guidance and in coaxial fashion a 22-gauge 3.5-inch spinal needle was advanced into the knee joint. Correct needle placement was confirmed by injecting a small amount of contrast and a knee joint arthrogram was obtained.

Disposition: The patient tolerated the procedure well without apparent complications. The patient was able to ambulate out of the facility in the same fashion they had entered. Discharge instructions were given.

Procedure name: Genicular Nerve Block

Diagnosis:

Consent: The risks, benefits and anticipated outcomes of the procedure, the risks and benefits of the alternatives to the procedure, and the roles and tasks of the personnel to be involved, were discussed with the patient. The patient has given written informed consent to the procedure and agrees to proceed.

Anesthesia:

Attending physician:

Assisting physician:

Patient information:

Procedure detail: The patient was brought into the procedure room and positioned supine on the fluoroscopy table with the affected knee flexed about 20 degrees supported with a pillow or foam. The affected knee was cleaned and draped in a sterile fashion. An anterior-posterior fluoroscopic view of the affected tibiofemoral joint was obtained with an open tibiofemoral joint space and equal width interspaces on both sides. The junctions connecting the femoral shaft to the superior lateral epicondyle and superior medial epicondyle, and the tibial shaft to the inferior medial epicondyle were marked separately. Skin and soft tissues were anesthetized with 1 mL 1% lidocaine. Under fluoroscopic guidance, total three 22-gauge 3.5-inch spinal needles with curved tip was advanced percutaneously towards areas connecting the shaft to the epicondyle, abutting the bone. A lateral fluoroscopic view was obtained, and needles were adjusted at the midline of the diaphysis and advanced to approximately 50-75% of the depth of femur. After negative aspiration, 2-3 ml of 0.25% bupivacaine was injected at each site. The needle was then restyletted and then removed with the tip intact. Hemostasis was easily achieved.

Disposition: The patient tolerated the procedure well without apparent complications. The patient was able to ambulate out of the facility in the same fashion they had entered. Discharge instructions were given.

Procedure name: Genicular Nerve Radiofrequency Ablation

Diagnosis:

Consent: The risks, benefits and anticipated outcomes of the procedure, the risks and benefits of the alternatives to the procedure, and the roles and tasks of the personnel to be involved, were discussed with the patient. The patient has given written informed consent to the procedure and agrees to proceed.

Anesthesia:

Attending physician:

Assisting physician:

Patient information:

Procedure detail: The patient was brought into the procedure room and positioned supine on the fluoroscopy table with the affected knee flexed about 20 degrees supported with a pillow or foam. The affected knee was cleaned and draped in a sterile fashion. An anterior-posterior fluoroscopic view of the affected tibiofemoral joint was obtained with an open tibiofemoral joint space and equal width interspaces on both sides. The junctions connecting the femoral shaft to the superior lateral epicondyle and superior medial epicondyle, and the tibial shaft to the inferior medial epicondyle were marked separately. Skin and soft tissues were anesthetized with 1 mL 1% lidocaine. Under fluoroscopic guidance, total three 22-gauge 3.5-inch radiofrequency needles with curved tip was advanced percutaneously towards areas connecting the shaft to the epicondyle, abutting the bone. A lateral fluoroscopic view was obtained, and needles were adjusted at the midline of the diaphysis and advanced to approximately 50-75% of the depth of femur. Sensory stimulation helped with the proximity of the needle tip to the nerve. Motor stimulation to 2 Hz was tested at all levels. Then, 90 seconds of 80-degree Celsius thermal radiofrequency ablation was performed at each level. The patient's knee was cleaned, and hemostasis was easily achieved.

Disposition: The patient tolerated the procedure well without apparent complications. The patient was able to ambulate out of the facility in the same fashion they had entered. Discharge instructions were given.

Procedure name: Femoral and obturator Nerve Block

Diagnosis:

Consent: The risks, benefits and anticipated outcomes of the procedure, the risks and benefits of the alternatives to the procedure, and the roles and tasks of the personnel to be involved, were discussed with the patient. The patient has given written informed consent to the procedure and agrees to proceed.

Anesthesia:

Attending physician:

Assisting physician:

Patient information:

Procedure detail: The patient was brought into the procedure room and positioned supine on the fluoroscopy table. The affected hip and groin area were cleansed and draped in sterile fashion. An anterior-posterior fluoroscopic view of the affected femoral-acetabular joint was obtained.

The track of the femoral nerve at 12 o'clock on the acetabulum and the track of the obturator nerve at the inferomedial border of the acetabulum were marked separately. Skin and soft tissues were anesthetized with 1 mL 1% lidocaine. Under fluoroscopic guidance, total two 23-gauge, 3.5-inch spinal needles were advanced percutaneously towards the above noted areas, until bone contact was made. After negative aspiration, 0.5 ml of contrast was injected to ensure placement outside the joint capsule and vasculature. After repeated negative aspiration, 1 ml of the solution containing 10 mg/ml and 1% lidocaine was injected to each site. The needle was then restyletted and then removed with the tip intact. Hemostasis was easily achieved.

Disposition: The patient tolerated the procedure well without apparent complications. The patient was able to ambulate out of the facility in the same fashion they had entered. Discharge instructions were given.

Procedure name: Intra-articular Hip Injection

Diagnosis:

Consent: The risks, benefits and anticipated outcomes of the procedure, the risks and benefits of the alternatives to the procedure, and the roles and tasks of the personnel to be involved, were discussed with the patient. The patient has given written informed consent to the procedure and agrees to proceed.

Anesthesia:

Attending physician:

Assisting physician:

Patient information:

Procedure detail: The patient was brought to the procedure room and positioned supine on the fluoroscopy table. Standard monitors were placed, and vital signs were observed. The affected area was cleaned and prepped in a sterile fashion. Using fluoroscopy, the femoral neck and greater trochanter were then identified and marked. The skin and subcutaneous tissues at this point were then anesthetized with 1% lidocaine using a 27-gauge, 1.5-inch needle. Then, a 23-gauge, 3.5-inch needle was directed toward the greater trochanter. On touching bone, the needle was retracted slightly, directed superiorly, and advanced to the junction of the femoral neck and femoral head. After negative aspiration, 0.5 mL of contrast was injected revealing an arthrogram. After repeated negative aspiration, 3-4 cc solution consisting of 10 mg/ml dexamethasone and 0.25% bupivacaine was easily injected. The needle was removed with the tip intact. Hemostasis was easily achieved.

Disposition: The patient tolerated the procedure well without apparent complications. The patient was able to ambulate out of the facility in the same fashion they had entered. Discharge instructions were given.

CHAPTER 7

SYMPATHETIC BLOCKS

SAM SCIRE, R.T., (R)(CT), ARRT, CRT
AND K.C. MAASUMI, M.D., M.S.

List of procedures in this chapter:

- Stellate Ganglion Block
- Celiac Plexus Block
- Lumbar Sympathetic Block
- Ganglion Impar Block
- Hypogastric Plexus Block

Procedure name: Stellate Ganglion Block

Diagnosis:

Consent: The risks, benefits and anticipated outcomes of the procedure, the risks and benefits of the alternatives to the procedure, and the roles and tasks of the personnel involved, were discussed with the patient. The patient has given written informed consent to the procedure and agrees to proceed.

Anesthesia:

Attending physician:

Assisting physician:

Patient information:

Procedure detail: The patient was transported into the procedure room and was positioned supine on the fluoroscopy table. A time-out was performed per the usual clinical fashion. Monitors were placed and vital signs were observed throughout the procedure. The patient's neck was slightly extended, prepped, and draped in a sterile manner. The C-arm was positioned in a true AP with the appropriate tilt to flatten the C6 endplates ipsilaterally. Using a radiopaque instrument, the skin overlying C5 and C7 were marked. The skin and subcutaneous tissues overlying C6 were anesthetized. Using two fingers, one over C5 and the other over C7, pressure was applied to retract the carotid artery laterally from the trachea. A 22-gauge spinal needle with a slight bend at the tip was advanced between the trachea and carotid artery and placed on the anterior tubercle of C6. Once bone was reached, the needle was pulled back 1-2 mm. After negative aspiration to rule out vascular return, contrast was injected under live fluoroscopy. AP and lateral views demonstrated a striated longitudinal spread and linear longitudinal spread, respectively. Absence of vascular uptake was also confirmed. A 10 ml mixture of 1% lidocaine and 0.5% bupivacaine was injected while performing intermittent negative aspirations to confirm the absence of vascular uptake. The needle was then removed, and hemostasis was achieved.

Disposition: The patient tolerated the procedure well without apparent complications. The patient was able to ambulate out of the facility in the same fashion they had entered. Discharge instructions were given.

After the procedure, look for the following: pain relief, change in temperature in the ipsilateral upper extremity, signs of Horner's Syndrome (ptosis, miosis, and anhidrosis), and redness of the conjunctiva.

Procedure name: Celiac Plexus Block

Diagnosis:

Consent: The risks, benefits and anticipated outcomes of the procedure, the risks and benefits of the alternatives to the procedure, and the roles and tasks of the personnel involved, were discussed with the patient. The patient has given written informed consent to the procedure and agrees to proceed.

Anesthesia:

Attending physician:

Assisting physician:

Patient information:

Procedure detail: The patient was transported into the procedure room and was positioned prone on the fluoroscopy table. A time-out was performed per the usual clinical fashion. Monitors were placed and vital signs were observed throughout the procedure. The patient's mid to lower back was prepped and draped in a sterile manner. The C-arm was positioned in an AP view with an appropriate tilt to flatten the L1 endplates. The C-arm was then obliqued to the patient's affected side until the tip of the transverse process was superimposed over the antero-lateral edge of the L1 vertebral body. The skin and subcutaneous tissues just lateral to the vertebral body and inferior to the transverse process were anesthetized. A 22-gauge 7-inch spinal needle with a slight bend at the tip was advanced towards the inferior/lateral edge of the L1 vertebral body until bone was reached. The C-arm was then positioned in a lateral view and the needle was navigated just anterior of the vertebral body. An AP view was checked to confirm placement in the middle of the mid-sagittal plane and the lateral border of the vertebral body. The C-arm was returned to a lateral view. After negative aspiration to rule out vascular return, contrast was injected under live fluoroscopy demonstrating a linear/longitudinal spread just anterior to vertebral body without vascular uptake. An AP view was then taken which demonstrated a striated longitudinal spread. The desired solution was injected. Using the same technique, the same procedure was performed on the patient's contralateral side. The needle was then removed, and hemostasis was achieved.

Disposition: The patient tolerated the procedure well without apparent complications. The patient was able to ambulate out of the facility in the same fashion they had entered. Discharge instructions were given.

Procedure name: Lumbar Sympathetic Block

Diagnosis:

Consent: The risks, benefits and anticipated outcomes of the procedure, the risks and benefits of the alternatives to the procedure, and the roles and tasks of the personnel involved, were discussed with the patient. The patient has given written informed consent to the procedure and agrees to proceed.

Anesthesia:

Attending physician:

Assisting physician:

Patient information:

Procedure detail: The patient was transported into the procedure room and was positioned prone on the fluoroscopy table. A positioning aid was used to reduce lumbar lordosis. A time-out was performed per the usual clinical fashion. Monitors were placed and vital signs were observed throughout the procedure. The patient's lower back was prepped and draped in a sterile manner. The C-arm was positioned in an AP view with an appropriate tilt to flatten the L3 endplates ipsilaterally. The C-arm was then obliqued to the patient's affected side until the tip of the transverse process was superimposed over the antero-lateral edge of the L3 vertebral body. The skin and subcutaneous tissues just lateral to the vertebral body and inferior to the transverse process were anesthetized. A 22-gauge 7-inch spinal needle with a slight bend at the tip was advanced towards the inferior/lateral edge of the L3 vertebral body until bone was reached. The C-arm was then positioned in a lateral view and the needle was navigated just anterior of the vertebral body. An AP view was checked to confirm placement in the middle of the mid-sagittal plane and the lateral border of the vertebral body. The C-arm was returned to a lateral view. After negative aspiration to rule out vascular return, contrast was injected under live fluoroscopy demonstrating a linear/longitudinal spread just anterior to vertebral body without vascular uptake. An AP view was then taken which demonstrated a striated longitudinal spread. The desired solution was injected. Using the same technique, the same procedure was performed on the patient's contralateral side. The needle was then removed, and hemostasis was achieved.

Disposition: The patient tolerated the procedure well without apparent complications. The patient was able to ambulate out of the facility in the same fashion they had entered. Discharge instructions were given.

Procedure name: Ganglion Impar Block

Diagnosis:

Consent: The risks, benefits and anticipated outcomes of the procedure, the risks and benefits of the alternatives to the procedure, and the roles and tasks of the personnel involved, were discussed with the patient. The patient has given written informed consent to the procedure and agrees to proceed.

Anesthesia:

Attending physician:

Assisting physician:

Patient information:

Procedure detail: The patient was transported into the procedure room and was positioned prone on the fluoroscopy table. A time-out was performed per the usual clinical fashion. Monitors were placed and vital signs were observed throughout the procedure. The patient's lower back and upper buttock area were prepped and draped in a sterile manner. The C-arm was positioned in a lateral view demonstrating an optimized view of the sacrococcygeal joint and the skin was marked. The C-arm was then positioned to an AP view and the sacrococcygeal joint was marked. The C-arm was returned to a lateral view. The overlying skin and subcutaneous tissues was anesthetized. Using a lateral view, a 22-gauge spinal needle was advanced through sacrococcygeal joint and positioned slightly anterior to the joint. After negative aspiration to rule out vascular return, contrast was injected under live fluoroscopy demonstrating a linear/longitudinal spread just anterior to the sacrum and without vascular uptake. An AP view was viewed demonstrating longitudinal contrast spread superimposed over the sacrococcygeal joint. The desired medication was injected. The needle was removed, and hemostasis was achieved.

Disposition: The patient tolerated the procedure well without apparent complications. The patient was able to ambulate out of the facility in the same fashion they had entered. Discharge instructions were given.

Procedure name: Hypogastric Plexus Block

Diagnosis:

Consent: The risks, benefits and anticipated outcomes of the procedure, the risks and benefits of the alternatives to the procedure, and the roles and tasks of the personnel involved, were discussed with the patient. The patient has given written informed consent to the procedure and agrees to proceed.

Anesthesia:

Attending physician:

Assisting physician:

Patient information:

Procedure detail: The patient was transported into the procedure room and was positioned prone on the fluoroscopy table. A time-out was performed per the usual clinical fashion. Monitors were placed and vital signs were observed throughout the procedure. The patient's back was prepped and draped in a sterile manner. The C-arm was positioned in an AP view with a cephalic tilt. The C-arm was obliqued towards the patient's affected side to form a direct path within a triangular window outlined by the transverse process, iliac crest, and the superior articulating process of the sacrum. The skin and subcutaneous tissues just lateral to the superior articulating process of the sacrum were anesthetized. A 22-gauge 7-inch spinal needle with a slight bend at the tip was advanced towards the inferior/lateral edge of the L5 vertebral body until bone was reached. The C-arm was then positioned in a lateral view and the needle was navigated just anterior of the vertebral body. An AP view was viewed to confirm placement in the middle of the mid-sagittal plane and the lateral border of the vertebral body. The C-arm was returned to a lateral view. After negative aspiration to rule out vascular return, contrast was injected under live fluoroscopy demonstrating a linear/longitudinal spread just anterior to vertebral body without vascular uptake. An AP view was then taken which demonstrated a longitudinal contrast spread superimposed over the L5 vertebral body. The desired solution was injected. Using the same technique, a second needle was placed on the patient's contralateral side. The needle was then removed, and hemostasis was achieved.

Disposition: The patient tolerated the procedure well without apparent complications. The patient was able to ambulate out of the facility in the same fashion they had entered. Discharge instructions were given.

CHAPTER 8

PERIPHERAL NERVE BLOCKS

K.C. MAASUMI, M.D., M.S.

List of Procedures in this chapter:

- Suprascapular Nerve Block (Ultrasound Guided)
- Subacromial bursa injection (Ultrasound Guided)
- Pudendal Nerve Block (Ultrasound Guided)
- Pudendal Nerve Block (Fluoroscopy Guided)
- Pudendal Nerve Radiofrequency Ablation (Fluoroscopy Guided)
- Saphenous Nerve Block (Ultrasound Guided)
- Ilioinguinal/Iliohypogastric Nerve Block (Ultrasound Guided)
- Ilioinguinal Nerve Pulsed Radiofrequency Ablation (Ultrasound Guided)
- Intercostal Nerve Block (Ultrasound Guided)
- Intercostal Nerve Block (Fluoroscopy Guided)
- Intercostal Nerve Pulsed Radiofrequency Ablation (Fluoroscopy Guided)
- Axillary Nerve Block (Ultrasound Guided)
- Tibial Nerve Block (Ultrasound Guided)
- Lateral Femoral Cutaneous Nerve Block (Ultrasound Guided)
- Obturator, Femoral, and Lateral Femoral Cutaneous Nerve Cooled Radiofrequency Ablation

Procedure name: Suprascapular Nerve Block (Ultrasound Guided)

Diagnosis:

Consent: The risks, benefits and anticipated outcomes of the procedure, the risks and benefits of the alternatives to the procedure, and the roles and tasks of the personnel involved, were discussed with the patient. The patient has given written informed consent to the Procedure and agrees to proceed.

Anesthesia:

Attending physician:

Assisting physician:

Patient information:

Procedure details: The patient was brought to the procedure room and placed in the sitting position. The area of the affected shoulder was prepped with Chlorhexidine and draped in a sterile manner. A linear ultrasound probe was draped with a sterile probe cover. Sonographic examination with sterile sonographic gel was performed in a coronal plane over the suprascapular fossa with a short axis to the line joining coracoid process and acromion (reflecting the position of the spinoglenoid notch). The skin and subcutaneous tissues at the targeted point were anesthetized with 1% lidocaine. A 22-gauge, 5-cm echogenic needle was advanced with ultrasound guidance until the needle tip landed in the spinoglenoid notch. After negative aspiration, a solution consisting of 1 cc of lidocaine and 1cc of 10mg/ml dexamethasone was injected. After the injection, the needle was removed with the tip intact. Hemostasis was easily achieved.

Disposition: The patient tolerated the procedure well without apparent complications. The patient was able to ambulate out of the facility in the same fashion they had entered. Discharge instructions were given.

Procedure name: Subacromial bursa injection (Ultrasound Guided)

Diagnosis:

Consent: The risks, benefits and anticipated outcomes of the procedure, the risks and benefits of the alternatives to the procedure, and the roles and tasks of the personnel involved, were discussed with the patient. The patient has given written informed consent to the procedure and agrees to proceed.

Anesthesia:

Attending physician:

Assisting physician:

Patient information:

Procedure detail: Patient is placed in the seated position. Ultrasound imaging of the subacromial bursa was used to place the transducer oriented in the coronal/scapular plane and positioned over the tip of the acromion. The bursa was identified as a thin anechoic fluid layer immediately above the tendon. Using a 25-gauge, 100mm echogenic needle, lidocaine was used as local anesthetic, then a solution containing 1 cc of lidocaine 1% and 1 cc of 10mg/ml dexamethasone was injected into the joint space without difficulty. The needle was removed, and hemostasis was achieved.

Disposition: The patient tolerated the procedure well without apparent complications. The patient was able to ambulate out of the facility in the same fashion they had entered. Discharge instructions were given.

Procedure name: Pudendal Nerve Block (Ultrasound Guided)

Diagnosis:

Consent: The risks, benefits and anticipated outcomes of the procedure, the risks and benefits of the alternatives to the procedure, and the roles and tasks of the personnel involved, were discussed with the patient. The patient has given written informed consent to the procedure and agrees to proceed.

Anesthesia:

Attending physician:

Assisting physician:

Patient information:

Procedure detail: The patient was brought into the procedure room and placed prone on the table. The area of interest was prepped with chlorhexidine and draped in a sterile manner. Using a linear ultrasound probe in a sterile sleeve, transverse view of the ilium was visualized. The probe was moved in a caudad direction until the iliac spine was visualized along with the pudendal nerve and artery. The skin and subcutaneous tissues in the area were anesthetized. A 3.5-inch 25-gauge spinal needle was advanced toward the pudendal nerve. After negative aspiration, hydro-dissection allowed to identify the pudendal nerve. A mixture of 10mg/ml of dexamethasone and 1% lidocaine was injected. The needle was then removed, and hemostasis was achieved.

Disposition: The patient tolerated the procedure well without apparent complications. The patient was able to ambulate out of the facility in the same fashion they had entered. Discharge instructions were given.

Procedure name: Pudendal Nerve Block (Fluoroscopy Guided)

Diagnosis:

Consent: The risks, benefits and anticipated outcomes of the procedure, the risks and benefits of the alternatives to the procedure, and the roles and tasks of the personnel involved, were discussed with the patient. The patient has given written informed consent to the procedure and agrees to proceed.

Anesthesia:

Attending physician:

Assisting physician:

Patient information:

Procedure detail: The patient was brought into the procedure room and placed prone on the fluoroscopy table. The area of the affected area was prepped with chlorhexidine and draped in a sterile manner. The ischial spine was identified under AP fluoroscopy with a slight caudal and slight ipsilateral oblique tilt. The skin and subcutaneous tissues in the area were anesthetized. A spinal needle was advanced toward the affected ischial spine until bone was contacted. The needle was then walked off bone medially. After negative aspiration, contrast was injected to confirm non-vascular needle tip location. After repeat negative aspiration, the desired solution was injected. The needle was then restyletted and fully removed with the tip intact. Hemostasis was easily achieved.

Disposition: The patient tolerated the procedure well without apparent complications. The patient was able to ambulate out of the facility in the same fashion they had entered. Discharge instructions were given.

Procedure name: Pudendal Nerve Radiofrequency Ablation (Fluoroscopy Guided)

Diagnosis:

Consent: The risks, benefits and anticipated outcomes of the procedure, the risks and benefits of the alternatives to the procedure, and the roles and tasks of the personnel involved, were discussed with the patient. The patient has given written informed consent to the Procedure and agrees to proceed.

Anesthesia:

Attending physician:

Assisting physician:

Patient information:

Procedure detail: The patient was brought into the procedure room and placed prone on the fluoroscopy table. The area of the affected area was prepped with chlorhexidine and draped in a sterile manner. The ischial spine was identified under AP fluoroscopy with a slight caudal and slight ipsilateral oblique tilt. The skin and subcutaneous tissues in the area were anesthetized. A RF needle was advanced toward the affected ischial spine until bone was contacted. The needle was then walked off bone medially. RF sensory stimulation was used to ensure proper needle tip location. During this part of the procedure, the patient identified sensory stimulation of the ipsilateral side of the genitalia. After, negative aspiration contrast was injected to confirm non-vascular needle tip location. After repeat negative aspiration, the desired solution was injected. The needle was then restyletted and fully removed with the tip intact. Hemostasis was easily achieved.

Disposition: The patient tolerated the procedure well without apparent complications. The patient was able to ambulate out of the facility in the same fashion they had entered. Discharge instructions were given.

Procedure name: Saphenous Nerve Block (Ultrasound Guided)

Diagnosis:

Consent: The risks, benefits and anticipated outcomes of the procedure, the risks and benefits of the alternatives to the procedure, and the roles and tasks of the personnel involved, were discussed with the patient. The patient has given written informed consent to the procedure and agrees to proceed.

Anesthesia:

Attending physician:

Assisting physician:

Patient information:

Procedure detail: The patient was brought to the procedure room and placed in the supine position on the table. A time-out was performed per the usual clinical fashion. Monitors were placed and vital signs were observed throughout the procedure. The area of interest was prepped with chlorhexidine and draped in a sterile manner. A linear ultrasound probe was draped with a sterile probe cover. Sonographic examination with sterile sonographic gel was utilized to reveal target nerve. The skin and subcutaneous tissues at the targeted point were anesthetized. A 22-gauge 5-cm needle was advanced with ultrasound guidance until the needle tip was visualized at the target site at approximately 2/3 down the thigh. Following negative aspiration, a 10 mL solution consisting of 1% lidocaine and 10mg/ml dexamethasone and preservative free normal saline was injected. After the injection, the needle was removed with the tip intact. Hemostasis was easily achieved.

Disposition: The patient tolerated the procedure well without apparent complications. The patient was able to ambulate out of the facility in the same fashion they had entered. Discharge instructions were given.

Procedure name: Ilioinguinal/Iliohypogastric Nerve Block (Ultrasound Guided)

Diagnosis:

Consent: The risks, benefits and anticipated outcomes of the procedure, the risks and benefits of the alternatives to the procedure, and the roles and tasks of the personnel involved, were discussed with the patient. The patient has given written informed consent to the procedure and agrees to proceed.

Anesthesia:

Attending physician:

Assisting physician:

Patient information:

Procedure detail: The patient was brought to the procedure room and placed supine on the table. Standard monitors were placed, and vital signs were observed throughout the procedure. The area of the abdomen was prepped and draped in a sterile manner. A linear ultrasound probe was draped with a sterile probe cover. Sonographic examination with sterile sonographic gel revealed the external oblique, internal oblique, and transversus abdominus muscle. The skin and subcutaneous tissues at the targeted point was anesthetized. A 25-gauge 3.5-cm needle was advanced with ultrasound guidance until the needle tip was visualized between the internal oblique and transversus abdominus muscles. Hydro-dissection was carried out with local anesthetic revealing the transversus abdominus plane. Then after negative aspiration, a solution consisting of 1% lidocaine and 10mg/ml dexamethasone was injected. After the injection, the needle was removed with the tip intact. Hemostasis was easily achieved.

Disposition: The patient tolerated the procedure well without apparent complications. The patient was able to ambulate out of the facility in the same fashion they had entered. Discharge instructions were given.

Procedure name: Ilioinguinal Nerve Pulsed Radiofrequency Ablation (Ultrasound Guided)

Diagnosis:

Consent: The risks, benefits and anticipated outcomes of the procedure, the risks and benefits of the alternatives to the procedure, and the roles and tasks of the personnel involved, were discussed with the patient. The patient has given written informed consent to the procedure and agrees to proceed.

Anesthesia:

Attending physician:

Assisting physician:

Patient information:

Procedure detail: The patient was brought to the procedure room and placed in the supine position on the table. Standard monitors were placed, and vital signs were observed throughout the procedure. The area of the affected lower abdomen was prepped with Chlorhexidine and draped in a sterile manner. A linear ultrasound probe was draped with a sterile probe cover. Sonographic examination with sterile sonographic gel was utilized to reveal the target. The skin and subcutaneous tissues at the targeted point were anesthetized. A 25-gauge 3.5-inch RF needle was advanced under ultrasound guidance until the needle tip was visualized. With intermittent negative aspiration, hydro dissection was carried out. Correct needle tip placement was verified with sensory stimulation at 50Hz and 0.5V. Then, pulsed radiofrequency was applied at 42C with cycles of 120 sec each. Afterwards, the needle was removed with the tip intact. Hemostasis was easily achieved.

Disposition: The patient tolerated the procedure well without apparent complications. The patient was able to ambulate out of the facility in the same fashion they had entered. Discharge instructions were given.

Procedure name: Intercostal Nerve Block (Ultrasound Guided)

Diagnosis:

Consent: The risks, benefits and anticipated outcomes of the procedure, the risks and benefits of the alternatives to the procedure, and the roles and tasks of the personnel involved, were discussed with the patient. The patient has given written informed consent to the procedure and agrees to proceed.

Anesthesia:

Attending physician:

Assisting physician:

Patient information:

Before positioning the patient, we marked the area of the patient's worse pain.

Procedure detail: The patient was brought into the procedure room and placed prone on the table. Standard monitors were placed, and vital signs were observed throughout the procedure. The area of the thorax was prepped and draped in a sterile manner. The area of most pain was identified with ultrasound, which correlated to the intercostal nerves aligning the affected ribs. The skin and subcutaneous tissues in these areas were anesthetized with. A 25-gauge, 3.5-inch spinal needle was directed toward the inferior aspect of each rib, using an in-plane approach. Careful attention was made to be clearly above the pleura. Once negative aspiration was confirmed, 1.5mL of a solution containing 1% lidocaine and 10mg/ml dexamethasone was injected.

Disposition: The patient tolerated the procedure well without apparent complications. The patient was able to ambulate out of the facility in the same fashion they had entered. Discharge instructions were given.

Procedure name: Intercostal Nerve Block (Fluoroscopy Guided)

Diagnosis:

Consent: The risks, benefits and anticipated outcomes of the procedure, the risks and benefits of the alternatives to the procedure, and the roles and tasks of the personnel involved, were discussed with the patient. The patient has given written informed consent to the Procedure and agrees to proceed.

Anesthesia:

Attending physician:

Assisting physician:

Patient information:

Procedure detail: The patient was brought into the procedure room and placed prone on the table. Standard monitors were placed, and vital signs were observed throughout the procedure. The area of the thorax was prepped and draped in a sterile manner. The area that is most painful was identified. The affected ribs and the inferior margin at the angle of each rib was identified under AP fluoroscopy. The skin and subcutaneous tissues in these areas were anesthetized. A 25-gauge, 1.5-inch needle was directed toward the inferior aspect of each rib under fluoroscopic guidance until the bone was contacted. From this point, the needle was walked off inferiorly. Once negative aspiration was confirmed, 1.5mL of a solution containing 1% lidocaine and 10mg/ml dexamethasone was injected.

Disposition: The patient tolerated the procedure well without apparent complications. The patient was able to ambulate out of the facility in the same fashion they had entered. Discharge instructions were given.

Procedure name: Intercostal Nerve Pulsed Radiofrequency Ablation (Fluoroscopy Guided)

Diagnosis:

Consent: The risks, benefits and anticipated outcomes of the procedure, the risks and benefits of the alternatives to the procedure, and the roles and tasks of the personnel involved, were discussed with the patient. The patient has given written informed consent to the procedure and agrees to proceed.

Anesthesia:

Attending physician:

Assisting physician:

Patient information:

Procedure detail: The patient was brought into the procedure room and placed prone on the table. Standard monitors were placed, and vital signs were observed throughout the procedure. The area of the thorax was prepped and draped in a sterile manner. The area that is most painful was identified. The affected ribs and the inferior margin at the angle of each rib was identified under AP fluoroscopy. The skin and subcutaneous tissues in these areas were anesthetized. An RF needle was directed toward the inferior aspect of the rib under fluoroscopic guidance until the bone was contacted. From this point, the needle was walked off inferiorly. Sensory stimulation was performed at 50 Hz, and we achieved sensory stimulation with patient confirming distribution of sensation in the painful region. Pulsed radiofrequency lesioning at 42 degrees Celsius for 120 seconds was performed. After lesioning, and after negative aspiration a desired solution was injected.

Disposition: The patient tolerated the procedure well without apparent complications. The patient was able to ambulate out of the facility in the same fashion they had entered. Discharge instructions were given.

Procedure name: Axillary Nerve Block (Ultrasound Guided)

Diagnosis:

Consent: The risks, benefits and anticipated outcomes of the procedure, the risks and benefits of the alternatives to the procedure, and the roles and tasks of the personnel involved, were discussed with the patient. The patient has given written informed consent to the Procedure and agrees to proceed.

Anesthesia:

Attending physician:

Assisting physician:

Patient information:

Procedure detail: The patient was brought into the procedure room and placed supine on the table. Standard monitors were placed, and vital signs were observed throughout the procedure. The area of the thorax was prepped and draped in a sterile manner. A linear ultrasound probe was draped with a sterile probe cover. An ultrasound survey image was obtained and he hyperechoic margin of the shaft of the humerus and the adjacent triceps muscle was identified. The transducer was then slowly moved toward the axilla while tracing the hyperechoic margin of the humerus until the hyperechoic margin curves outward as the transducer approached the inferior head of the humerus. Below the point of this outward curve lies the axillary nerve and posterior circumflex humeral artery. A 22-gauge, 5-cm echogenic needle was advanced with ultrasound guidance until the needle tip landed in the desired location as described above. Then the desired solution was injected. After the injection, the needle was removed with the tip intact. Hemostasis was easily achieved.

Disposition: The patient tolerated the procedure well without apparent complications. The patient was able to ambulate out of the facility in the same fashion they had entered. Discharge instructions were given.

Procedure name: Tibial Nerve Block (Ultrasound Guided)

Diagnosis:

Consent: The risks, benefits and anticipated outcomes of the procedure, the risks and benefits of the alternatives to the procedure, and the roles and tasks of the personnel involved, were discussed with the patient. The patient has given written informed consent to the procedure and agrees to proceed.

Anesthesia:

Attending physician:

Assisting physician:

Patient information:

Procedure detail: The patient was brought into the procedure room and placed supine on the table with the lower extremity slightly frog legged. Standard monitors were placed, and vital signs were observed throughout the procedure. The area of the thorax was prepped and draped in a sterile manner. A linear ultrasound probe was draped with a sterile probe cover. Sonographic examination with sterile sonographic gel was utilized to reveal the affected tibial vessels at the level slightly above the medial malleolus, and the tibial nerve. The skin and subcutaneous tissues at the targeted point were anesthetized. A 30-gauge 1-inch needle was advanced with ultrasound guidance in an out of plane approach until the needle tip was visualized at the posterior edge of the tibial nerve. Then after negative aspiration, the desired solution was injected. After the injection, the needle was removed with the tip intact. Hemostasis was easily achieved.

Disposition: The patient tolerated the procedure well without apparent complications. The patient was able to ambulate out of the facility in the same fashion they had entered. Discharge instructions were given.

Procedure name: Lateral Femoral Cutaneous Nerve Block (Ultrasound Guided)

Diagnosis:

Consent: The risks, benefits and anticipated outcomes of the procedure, the risks and benefits of the alternatives to the procedure, and the roles and tasks of the personnel involved, were discussed with the patient. The patient has given written informed consent to the procedure and agrees to proceed.

Anesthesia:

Attending physician:

Assisting physician:

Patient information:

Procedure detail: The patient was brought to the procedure room and placed in the supine position on the fluoroscopy table. Standard monitors were placed, and vital signs were observed throughout the procedure. The area of the abdomen was prepped and draped in a sterile manner. A linear ultrasound probe was draped with a sterile probe cover. Sonographic examination with sterile sonographic gel revealed the sartorius muscle and lateral femoral cutaneous nerve superior and lateral to the sartorius muscle. The skin and subcutaneous tissues at the targeted point was anesthetized. A spinal needle was advanced with ultrasound guidance until the needle tip was visualized along the lateral border of the sartorius muscle and lateral femoral cutaneous nerve. Then after negative aspiration, the desired solution was injected. After the injection, the needle was removed with the tip intact. Hemostasis was easily achieved.

Disposition: The patient tolerated the procedure well without apparent complications. The patient was able to ambulate out of the facility in the same fashion they had entered. Discharge instructions were given.

Procedure name: Obturator, Femoral, and Lateral Femoral Cutaneous Nerve Cooled Radiofrequency Ablation

Diagnosis:

Consent: The risks, benefits and anticipated outcomes of the procedure, the risks and benefits of the alternatives to the procedure, and the roles and tasks of the personnel involved, were discussed with the patient. The patient has given written informed consent to the procedure and agrees to proceed.

Anesthesia:

Attending physician:

Assisting physician:

Patient information:

Procedure detail: The patient was brought to the procedure room and placed in the supine position on the fluoroscopy table. Standard monitors were placed, and vital signs were observed. A universal protocol timeout was conducted in the usual fashion. Under AP view, the femoral head and acetabulum were identified and marked. The skin and subcutaneous tissues at this point were then anesthetized. An RF needle was directed toward the location of the obturator nerve, inferior to the inferomedial edge of the hip joint, along the ischium to the inferior incisura. Bone was contacted, sensory and motor testing were performed. After negative aspiration was confirmed, contrast was used to confirm non vascular needle tip location. Then, the area over the acetabulum at the 12 o'clock and 10 o'clock position of the femoral head was marked for the location of the femoral and lateral femoral cutaneous nerves, and the skin anesthetized at a point lateral and inferior to the inguinal crease. Then an RF needle was directed toward these two locations. When bone was contacted, sensory and motors testing was done. After negative aspiration was confirmed, lesioning was performed. The needle was then restyletted and then removed with the tip intact. Hemostasis was easily achieved.

Disposition: The patient tolerated the procedure well without apparent complications. The patient was able to ambulate out of the facility in the same fashion they had entered. Discharge instructions were given.

CHAPTER 9

INFUSION THERAPY

K.C. MAASUMI, M.D., M.S.

Introduction:

Infusion therapy utilizes a variety of different medications. It is important to learn about the side effects of the medications being used and be cautiously and meticulously when using them concomitantly with the other medications that the patient is taking.

Prior to infusion therapy, patient is required to have completed basic labs including BMP, CBC, LFT, and an ECG. It is prudent to have a baseline information about the labs so that changes during and after the infusion can be assessed and evaluated properly.

Infusion therapy is meant mainly for intractable chronic pain including intractable chronic migraine, complex regional pain syndrome (CRPS), and several other chronic pain syndromes. There are books dedicated to infusion therapy; however, this chapter touches on the basics of some of the medications that can be infused, and it is not meant to be a comprehensive discussion of infusion therapy.

Chronic migraine

There are patients whose headaches do not attenuate with oral or even injectable medications. You will have to know the patient's past history very well before considering infusion therapy. At some centers the infusion therapy is done as an inpatient admission and at other centers it is done as an outpatient admission. The key to a successful outcome is doing the infusion in multiple doses over the course of a week using the medication of choice. Most patients will not have any meaningful outcome if they are infused only once.

Information regarding Valproate infusion

Valproate is a medication that has been used for decades to treat chronic headaches. Studies have shown that intravenous (IV) Valproate infusion is a safe and well tolerated medication for the treatment of chronic migraine resistant to oral medications. The goal of inpatient IV Valproate treatment is to break the cycle of headache with repetitive doses.

Pre-admission clearance

In order to be cleared for admission, the patient must complete basic labs such as CBC, BMP, LFT, and ECG. These tests must be reviewed at least a week prior to admission in order to allow ample time for adjustments.

Preparing for the Hospitalization

There should be a pre-admission visit to review all home medications. The patient must maintain good hydration before and during hospitalization.

What to expect during your stay?

During the hospital stay, Valproate will be administered intravenously approximately every eight hours.

What side effects should be expected?

Side effects may include dizziness, headache, changes in taste, and sleepiness. Liver and ammonia level are monitored to ensure the safe continuation of infusions. Liver toxicity and elevated blood ammonia levels are rare, but possible adverse effects of IV Valproate. If there is any indication of increased or unsafe levels in the blood, skip a dose and monitor the levels. If they remain high, then it is best to stop the infusions.

Headaches may occur intermittently during the hospitalization while being infused. Patients are advised to keep a headache diary to track nausea and headache levels during the stay. It is best to avoid acute headache treatment while receiving IV Valproate infusion in order for it to work optimally. Patient may be reluctant to skip acute medications; however, they should try their best effort to minimize the use of various medications at the same time.

What happens after the hospitalization?

While IV Valproate is not a cure for migraine, most patients will achieve thc goal of a reduction in frequency and severity of their headaches for weeks to months after discharge.

Many patients may still have headaches at the time of discharge. It may take two weeks to a month following the hospital stay before the maximum improvement occurs. Headache freedom at discharge is not predictive of the overall benefit from IV Valproate. Prior to discharge, develop a headache care plan with the patient.

How to infuse Valproate

Valproate 500-1000 mg/5 ml in 50 cc NS- Infused over 20 min

Information regarding IV Dihydroergotamine (DHE)

Dihydroergotamine (DHE) is a medication from the ergotamine family and is a distant relative of the triptan class of medications (i.e., sumatriptan, naratriptan, almotriptan, rizatriptan, frovatriptan, eletriptan and zolmitriptan). DHE is generally well tolerated and very helpful to many patients with frequent headache. DHE has been used for headache for over 50 years. Inpatient treatment with IV DHE has been an established practice for over 20 years and is endorsed by the American Academy of Neurology. The goal of inpatient DHE treatment is to break the cycle of headache with repetitive doses.

Pre-admission clearance

In order to be cleared for admission, the patient must complete basic labs such as CBC, BMP, LFT, and ECG. These tests must be reviewed at least a week prior to admission in order to allow ample time for adjustments.

Preparing for the Hospitalization

There should be a pre-admission visit to review all home medications. The patient must maintain good hydration before and during hospitalization. Review all home medications. Make sure the patient is not taking any triptans within 24 hours of admission. Examples of some triptans are sumatriptan, naratriptan, almotriptan, rizatriptan, frovatriptan, eletriptan and zolmitriptan.

What to expect during the hospitalization

During the hospitalization, DHE will be administered intravenously every eight hours. The dose will be increased over the first three doses, allowing for adjustments depending on the patient's response. The most common side effect of DHE is nausea. Provide anti-nausea medications to the patient prior to each dose of DHE. Other common side effects include stomach cramping, leg cramping, and diarrhea.

In a small number of patients, their headaches may briefly worsen after the first few doses of DHE. This side effect is generally short lived and improves after a few doses of infusion. However, if the headache becomes intolerable during the treatment, slowing the rate of administration can resolve this side effect.

Advise patient to keep a headache diary to track nausea and headache levels during the hospitalization. It is best to go without other acute headache treatment medications while receiving DHE for it to work optimally.

What happens after the hospitalization?

While IV DHE is not a cure for migraine, most patients will achieve the goal of a reduction in their headaches for weeks to months after discharge. Many patients still have headaches at the time of discharge. It may take four to six weeks following the hospital stay before the maximum improvement occurs. Headache freedom at discharge is not predictive of the overall benefit from IV DHE.

How to infuse DHE

- 0.25 mg × 4 placed in four ¼ dose bags in 50 cc NS; each ¼ dose bag infused over 20 min
- 0.50 mg × 2 placed in two ½ dose bags of NS; each ½ dose bag infused over 30 min
- 1 mg placed in 50 cc NS infused over 30 min

Lidocaine infusion:

It is imperative that the lidocaine infusion is done in the hospital inpatient setting due to its variety of adverse effects. Lidocaine can be infused at 1g in a 250 ml 5% glucose solution. Infusion rate is 1-4 mg/min (maximum rate is 3.4mg/kg/hr or 0.0567 mg/kg/min). Start at 1 mg/min and titrate up until headache improves.

Prior to infusion resting EKG and liver function test must be monitored: any previously known hypokalemia should be corrected. During the infusion, patient should have continuous cardiac monitoring at least every 30 minutes looking for cardiac arrhythmias.

Adverse Effects:

- Bradycardia, cardiac arrhythmias, and hypotension.
- Sensation of heat or cold, numbness, paresthesia, nystagmus, twitching, and tremor are signs of high plasma levels of lidocaine.
- Convulsions, cardiovascular collapse, and respiratory arrest are symptoms of an overdose. (Plasma concentration of more than 9mg/L.)
- Nausea and vomiting
- Psychiatric symptoms including paranoid ideation may be triggered and the infusion should be stopped.

Contraindications:

- Cardiac arrhythmia, Pregnancy, and lactation.
- Epilepsy, peptic ulcers, psychiatric disease.

Note, if the patient is taking propranolol or cimetidine, the clearance of lidocaine may be reduced causing lidocaine toxicity.

Other medications that can be infused concomitantly with the above medication:

- Dexamethasone 10 mg in 50 cc NS- infused over 20 min
- Prochlorperazine 10 mg/2 ml in 50 cc NS- infused over 20 min
- Diphenhydramine 25- 50 mg 2-5 min IV push
- Metoclopramide 10 mg/2 ml in 50 cc NS- Infused over 20 min
- Methocarbamol 1 gm in 50 cc NS- Infused over 20 min
- Ondansetron 8mg/ml in 50 cc NS- Infused over 30 min
- Levetiracetam 500 mg/5 ml in 100 cc NS- Infused over 20 min
- Ketorolac 30 mg/2-5 min IV push
- Methylprednisolone 500-1000 mg in 250 cc NS- Infused over 1 hour
- Magnesium sulfate1-2 gm in 250 cc NS- Infuse1 hour
- Diazepam 2.5-5 mg in 50 cc NS- Infused over 20 min
- Famotidine 20 mg in 50 cc NS- Infused over 20 min

CHAPTER 10

CLINICAL NOTES

WILLIAM QUBTY, MD
AND K.C. MAASUMI, M.D., M.S.

Introduction:

As a mentor once wisely instructed, a pain history is taken, not given. Pain is multifactorial and requires a thorough understanding of its nuances to obtain the correct diagnosis while limiting unnecessary and invasive testing. Thus, the clinician must be able to ask open ended questions yet direct the patient when needed to obtain a comprehensive and succinct history. History is best obtained from the person experiencing the symptoms if they are able. The patient should be asked to sit closest to the clinician, if others are present, to minimize distractions. Oftentimes, eager family members want to contribute to the history, but the clinician should encourage the patient to report their symptoms in their own words. Building patient rapport takes time, and history taking is typically best done sitting with the patient in a calm manner when possible.

Establishing the timeline of pain is crucial to diagnosis and management. It is important to know when the pain began and when it worsened. The circumstances of its onset are necessary in understanding if the pain is due to a primary or secondary disorder. For example, in a new onset persistent headache, the clinician should ask about preceding illness, travel to high altitude, head trauma, new medication use, recreational drug use, heavy lifting, or excessive Valsalva.

When asking about pain frequency and duration, we should discuss not only when pain is bothersome but when it is present and to what degree. For example, when interviewing patients with low back pain, it is important to determine if the pain has been present for less than 6 weeks (acute) 6-12 weeks (subacute), or greater than 12 weeks (chronic) as most back pain may resolve with time. The clinician should understand if the pain is stable, improving or worsening over time. A bonus would be if we can find out how the pain is affecting patient's activities of daily living.

The location of the pain and if the pain radiates to other areas should also be discussed in detail. The quality of the pain whether sharp, dull, achy, electrical, or throbbing is useful information. For example, radicular symptoms originating from a lumbar herniated disc may be described as an electrical shooting pain that starts in the low back and travels down into the lower extremity. Sometimes, if patients can help understand the pattern of radiation, the clinician can even make an educated guess which nerve roots might be affected. Some of the associated symptoms in patients with cervical or lumbar radiculopathy include numbness, tingling or even weakness in dermatomal distribution.

Migraine pain may be described as a unilateral throbbing sensation. On the other hand, neck pain that radiates from the back of the head forward, may indicate cervicogenic headache. The location and quality of pain could also suggest a somatic referred pain such as cervical pain referring to the area between the scapulae.

The associated features of pain are also important to characterize. For example, in assessing headache disorders, commonly associated migrainous symptoms include photophobia, phonophobia, osmophobia, nausea, emesis, movement sensitivity, lightheadedness, tinnitus and vertigo. Aura is a reversible and typically self-limiting neurologic symptom and occurs in one quarter to one third of people with migraine. Aura may occur prior to or during the headache phase of migraine. The clinician should query the patient if there are any associated progressive visual changes, paresthesia, speech impairments, motor weakness, ataxia, or alteration in level of awareness.

Cranial autonomic features are common in primary headache disorders; they are usually bilateral in migraine, if present, and unilateral in cluster headache. Cranial autonomic features include periorbital discoloration or edema, ptosis, conjunctival injection, lacrimation, rhinorrhea, aural fullness, facial diaphoresis, or facial flushing.

Pain triggers or exacerbating factors are an essential part of the history. For migraine, common potential triggers include menses, high altitude, bright lights, loud sounds, strong smells, dehydration, fasting, let down from stress, change in sleep schedule and excessive screen time (Table 1). Migraine triggers should not be confused with premonitory symptoms which are quite common. Premonitory symptoms precede the headache phase of migraine and are believed to involve the hypothalamus and limbic regions. Thus, the symptoms include change in appetite, yawning, fatigue, light and sound sensitivity, polyuria, and mood change. Flexion can trigger radicular pain, extension can trigger facetogenic pain.

Table 1: Common Potential Migraine Triggers

Menses	Excessive physical activity
High altitude	Bright lights
Loud sounds	Strong odors
Hot weather	Barometric pressure change
Dehydration	Fasting
Stress	Let down from stress
Change in sleep duration	Excessive screen time

Red flag features of pain vary based on the location or type of pain. For headaches, concerning features include headache worsening immediately upon standing and improving upon lying down. This suggests CSF hypovolemia and/or leak. Headaches that regularly awaken patients from sleep suggest increased intracranial pressure. Timing of pain reaching maximal intensity is also useful. For example, if a patient presents with a severe headache with explosive or thunderclap onset, this typically warrants urgent work up to rule out intracranial hemorrhage. For back pain, it is important to query if there are neurologic signs or symptoms in the corresponding upper or lower extremities. For example, with low back pain, red flag signs and symptoms include bowel/bladder dysfunction or incontinence, saddle anesthesia, weakness in the lower extremities, constitutional symptoms, or fever. A pain focused review of systems is illustrated in Table 2.

Table 2: Pain Focused Review of Systems

Constitutional	Weight loss, fever, chills, fatigue
Head, Ears, Eyes, Nose, Throat	Vision loss, diplopia, hearing loss
Skin	Rash, color change, congenital lesions
Cardiovascular	Chest pain, palpitations
Pulmonary	Shortness of breath, cough
Gastrointestinal	Nausea, vomiting, diarrhea, rectal bleeding
Genitourinary	Dysuria, incontinence, pregnancy
Neurological	Dizziness, syncope, ataxia, paresthesia
Musculoskeletal	Joint pain, swelling, erythema, back pain
Hematologic	Easy bruising, prolonged bleeding
Endocrinologic	Cold or heat intolerance, excess sweating, menstrual irregularity
Psychiatric	Anxiety, depression, mood change, suicidal ideation

The level of disability due to pain should be discussed. Disability can be illustrated qualitatively by asking if pain is mild, moderate, or severe. The patient should discuss how the pain impacts their physical, emotional, cognitive, financial and relationship well-being. Quantitatively there are validated surveys for headache disability such as the Migraine Disability Assessment (MIDAS) and the Headache Impact Test-6 (HIT-6). These quantitative assessments are also helpful to complete during follow up visits to monitor treatment efficacy.

Inquire what alleviates the pain. Current and prior pain treatments including pharmacologic, non-pharmacologic and interventional procedures should be queried. The clinician should be aware of the dose, frequency, benefit, and adverse effects of each treatment, medication allergies as well as past medical history to better assess treatment contraindications. All prior relevant diagnostic data including laboratory testing and imaging should be reviewed.

Pain may have a genetic component and thus a family history of pain disorders should be obtained. Common genetic-associated pain disorders include migraine, certain neuropathies, fibromyalgia, and connective tissue disorders such as Ehlers-Danlos syndrome and ankylosing spondylitis. In patients with headache, it is important to ask about family history of aneurysms.

Below is a sample complete note template for a new patient consultation.

Thank you for referring [Name], a [age] year old, [Handedness gender] who I saw at [Clinic] in consultation for headache, as requested by ***.

Headache history:

Headaches began at age *** and became more bothersome at age ***. There was/was not preceding illness, travel to high altitude, head trauma, new medication, recreational drug use, or constipation/heavy lifting/excessive Valsalva.

Currently, headache occurs *** days per month. This has been the pattern for ***. Severe headache occurs *** days per month. The onset of headache to peak is ***. These headaches typically last *** hours and can last up to ***.

The pain is located in *** and has a *** quality.

Associated symptoms include photophobia, phonophobia, osmophobia, nausea, emesis, non-pulsatile tinnitus, movement sensitivity, neck stiffness, lightheadedness, vertigo

There is/is not a diurnal or positional variation. It does not worsen with cough, Valsalva, or bending over and there are no regular overnight awakenings due to headache. There is/is not an associated diplopia.

There are/are not visual, motor, sensory, language, or brainstem aura symptoms.

Premonitory phase symptoms include: yawning, fatigue, neck pain, excessive urination, mood changes, food cravings

There are/are not cranial autonomic symptoms (Cranial autonomic symptoms include ptosis, periorbital edema or color change, conjunctival injection, lacrimation, nasal congestion or discharge, aural fullness, facial flushing, facial pallor, facial diaphoresis)

Triggers include photophobia, phonophobia, osmophobia, nausea, emesis, movement sensitivity, neck stiffness, tinnitus, lightheadedness, and vertigo.

Patient is planning to become pregnant/breastfeeding: Yes or No

MIDAS: ***

HIT6: ***

Current medications:

Prior Treatments: List them and then ask the patient which of the previously tried medications worked well, did not work, or could not tolerate due to severe side effects.

Preventive medications:

CGRP antagonists: erenumab, fremanezumab, galcanezumab, eptinezumab, atogepant, rimegepant (every other day use)

Antihypertensives:

Beta-blockers: Propranolol, nadolol, atenolol, metoprolol, timolol
Calcium channel blockers: verapamil, diltiazem, nifedipine, amlodipine
ACE inhibitors: lisinopril
Angiotensin Receptor Blockers: Candesartan
Antiepileptics: gabapentin, Pregabalin, topiramate, valproic acid

Antidepressants:

Tricyclics: amitriptyline, nortriptyline, doxepin, imipramine, protriptyline, desipramine
SNRIs: Venlafaxine, duloxetine, desvenlafaxine
SSRIs: Fluoxetine, sertraline, paroxetine, fluvoxamine, citalopram, escitalopram

MAO inhibitors: phenelzine, tranylcypromine
Norepinephrine and dopamine reuptake inhibitor: bupropion

Anxiolytics: Buspirone

Serotonin antagonists: Cyproheptadine, Ergotamine

Herbal, vitamins, and mineral supplements: Riboflavin (Vitamin B2, Coenzyme Q10 (CoQ10), Magnesium glycinate, Feverfew

Others: oxygen, lithium, acetaminophen, OnabotulinumtoxinA injections, greater/lesser occipital nerve block, acupuncture, massage therapy, physical therapy, chiropractic manipulation, pain psychology sessions.

Abortive medications:
CGRP antagonist: ubrogepant, rimegepant
5HT3 antagonists: Ondansetron
Antihistamines: Diphenhydramine, metoclopramide, Hydroxyzine, Meclizine
Barbiturates: Butalbital/Acetaminophen/Caffeine
Ergots: dihydroergotamine
NSAIDs: Naproxen, ketorolac, indomethacin, Excedrin, ibuprofen, ketoprofen, diclofenac, meloxicam, celecoxib, Nabumetone
Steroids: prednisone
Triptans: Naratriptan, almotriptan, frovatriptan, sumatriptan, rizatriptan, eletriptan, zolmitriptan

Prior imaging and other pertinent testing:

Relevant Past Medical and Surgical History:

Allergies:

Social history:

Family history
Migraine or other headaches in the family
Aneurysms in a first degree relative

Review of systems

CONSTITUTIONAL: weight loss, fever, chills, weakness, fatigue
HEENT: visual loss, double vision, hearing loss, snoring
SKIN: rashes

CARDIOVASCULAR: chest pain, palpitations, myocardial infarctions
PULMONARY: shortness of breath, cough
GASTROINTESTINAL: nausea, vomiting, diarrhea
GENITOURINARY: burning on urination
NEUROLOGICAL: dizziness, syncope, ataxia, numbness, tingling, weakness
MUSCULOSKELETAL: joint pain, back pain, neck pain
HEMATOLOGIC: bleeding issues, bruising
PSYCHIATRIC: anxiety, depression
ENDOCRINOLOGIC: sweating

General examinations:

Vitals:

General: appearance of patient
HEENT: point of tenderness, allodynia, temporal pulses, fundoscopy
Skin: rashes or lesions
Lungs: breathing labored or not, whether patient is wheezing
Cardiac exam: rate, rhythm of heart
Vascular: cyanosis, edema, or carotid bruits
Abdominal: tenderness or masses; look for hernias
Extremities: Circulation, pitting edema
Musculoskeletal: gross deformities

Neurological exam:

Mental Status:
Alertness and orientation of the patient to place and time.
Affect and speech

Cranial Nerves:
II –Visual fields
III, IV, VI – movement of the extra-ocular muscle movement, pupillary reactions to light
V – facial sensation to light touch
VII – symmetry of the face
VIII – hearing
IX, X – movement of the palate
XI – strength of the sternocleidomastoid
XII – movement of the tongue

Motor Exam: address the following:
Bulk: whether there is atrophy or not
Strength:

	Delt	Biceps	Triceps	Wrist Ext	Wrist Flex	Finger Flex	Finger Ext	Finger Abd	Finger Add
Right	5/5	5/5	5/5	5/5	5/5	5/5	5/5	5/5	5/5
Left	5/5	5/5	5/5	5/5	5/5	5/5	5/5	5/5	5/5

	Hip Flex	Hip Ext	BiFem (knee flex)	Quads (knee ext)	Gastroc (plantflx)	TibAnt (Dorsiflx)	TibPost (ank add)
Right	5/5	5/5	5/5	5/5	5/5	5/5	5/5
Left	5/5	5/5	5/5	5/5	5/5	5/5	5/5

Sensation: Whether sensation to light touch, vibration, and temperature are normal; Romberg testing

Cerebellar: Ataxia, tremor, movement of the finger to nose, heel to shin and rapid alternating movements

Reflexes:
Hoffman sign

	Right	Left
Bicep	2/4	2/4
Triceps	2/4	2/4
BrRad	2/4	2/4
Knee	2/4	2/4
Ankle	2/4	2/4

Gait: Patient's gait and whether patient is able to do heel, toe, and tandem walks

MSK:

Cervical spine:

Visual: no visible deformity, no overlying rash
Flexion:
Extension:
Rotation:
Paraspinal tenderness or palpable trigger points:
Cervical facet loading maneuvers reproduces symptoms:

Assessment:

[Patient name] is a *** year old [male/female] with a history of *** presenting for evaluation of headache. The most likely diagnosis is ***. Comment on the image findings; comment on examination; comment on relevant past medical, surgical, and family history; state your differential diagnoses and which one you think is most likely than not to be the cause of the present illness.

Recommendations:

- Conservative therapy:
  - Physical therapy
  - Chiropractic treatments
  - Acupuncture
  - Pain psychology
  - Over the counter medications such as NSAIDs
- Acute treatment options:
- Preventive trial options:
- Necessary diagnostic tests:
  - XR, MRI, CT, EMG/NCS, EEG etc.

For more advanced treatment options, like OnabotulinumtoxinA injections, clinicians may have to explain what preventive treatments patients has tried: The patient has tried antiepileptic drugs (list 1-2 medications), antihypertensive drugs (list 1-2 medications), and antidepressants (list 1-2 medications) each longer than 3 months without significant benefit. Explain the frequency of headaches; for example, there are more than 15 headaches per month, 8 of which are migrainous. The next step is OnabotulinumtoxinA injections per.

It is widely accepted that migraine involves activation and sensitization of trigeminovascular pathways. Patients with intractable chronic migraine would benefit from blocking the pathways at multiple junctures. For this reason, in addition to the OnabotulinumtoxinA injections every 12 weeks, nerve blocks can be used such as Greater and Lesser Occipital Nerve Block (to modulate the trigeminal pathway via the C2 and C3 nerve roots) as well as Sphenopalatine Ganglion (SPG) Block. The SPG is composed of branches of V2 and some V1 of the trigeminal nerve and has both sympathetic and parasympathetic nerve fibers which are activated in chronic migraine. It would be most efficacious to perform these nerve blocks every 4 to 6 weeks between the OnabotulinumtoxinA treatments.

If the patient is female and of childbearing age, then please discuss cessation of any medications that would potentially cause harm to the growing fetus. It is best to refer the patient to her obstetrician to have a more in-depth discussion. Further discuss that smoking and high dose hormone replacement, in setting of migraine with aura may increase the risk of stroke.

Further, discuss smoking, birth control pills or any hormone replacement will increase the risk of stroke in patients with migraine, especially in those with an aura.

Lifestyle changes

Regularity of daily schedule is important; regular sleep, regular exercise, regular meals, and maintaining good hydration

When headache is more severe, changes in immediate environment can help alleviate the pain. For example limiting stimuli by doing things like turning off the lights and going to a quiet room can be helpful. If sleep is possible, sleep can sometimes be helpful. Limit use of medications such as ibuprofen and acetaminophen to 3 or fewer days per week.